Rob Shickel

I0103991

Cancer:
My Cancer Never Sleeps!

Part Two of Putting the How Into Hope
.... to Change Certainty

1st Edition

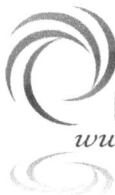

MY CHRONIC CANCER
www.mychroniccancer.com

Cancer: My Cancer Never Sleeps!

Author/Publisher's Note
This book is a novel and, therefore, it is a work of fiction. All names, all characters, all places and all incidents as used herein are fictitious and the product(s) of the author's imagination. Any resemblance to actual events, to places or to persons, whether living or dead, is entirely coincidental.

Published in the USA by My Chronic Cancer LLC
Shickel, Robert
Cancer: My Cancer Never Sleeps! / Robert Shickel – 1st ed.

ISBN 978-0-9887273-2-8
Library of Congress Cataloging-in-Publication Data: Robert Shickel, My Cancer Never Sleeps, Chronic Cancer, Cancer Advocacy, DNA-like Framework.

Printed in the United States

* * * * * * *

... in cancer our real goal is to change certainty.
- Rob Shickel

Other Works on My Chronic Cancer™ by Rob Shickel

- *Cancer: Who Gave Me Cancer?©*
  Part One of Putting the How Into Hope™
  Companion to Cancer My Cancer Never Sleeps©

- *Cancer: My Chronic Cancer Strategy©*
  Part Three of Putting the How Into Hope™
  Creating and maintaining a cancer-offensive strategy

- *Cancer: My Cancer Advocacy Tactics©*
  Part Four of Putting the How Into Hope™
  Cancer tactics to achieve My Cancer Advocacy™

- *Cancer: My Chronic Cancer Agenda To-Do List©*
  Part Five of Putting the How Into Hope™
  Create and maintain a cancer-centric to-do list™

- Cancer: Characters©
  Part Six of Putting the How Into Hope™
  Chronic Cancer Advocates and their stories™

Fiction by Rob Shickel
- Shadowing Beacon©

FYI: Why Are We Here?

Cancer: My Cancer Never Sleeps© is Part Two of Putting the How into Hope™ for cancer patients world-wide. Our goal is that this book become a kind of reference and methodology for cancer patients, as "What did he do?", "Why did his oncologist do that?", and "I didn't know I could do that …"

Cancer: My Cancer Never Sleeps© is intentionally gender neutral. It deals with indolent and aggressive cancers, and with curable and incurable cancers as they would apply to both genders.

The journey of our three cancer patients has been divided into two volumes.

• First, Cancer: Who Gave Me Cancer?© deals with the news of just having been diagnosed with cancer. We experience the patient's initial reactions, cancer treatments and making/not-making sense in the midst of chaos. Think "boot camp" and foundation building in the context of your cancer.

Here is where we build the foundation, the basement and the essential supporting infra-structure. In doing so we focus on the twin goals of cancer as a chronic condition (strategic goal) and on the development of our own cancer advocacy (tactics).

• Second, Cancer: My Cancer Never Sleeps© extends the My Chronic Cancer Advocacy methodology for each patient into cancer's harsh realities without pulling punches. Think "build-out" with re-useable tools to counter-attack cancer as an adversary, to re-gain our health and to return to a reasonably normal life. After all, cancer doesn't soften the blow or pull punches. You shouldn't either.

Also, by intent, neither book attempts to be a complete source on the cancer experience. This is because cancer will be experienced differently due to the cancer, by religion, ethnicity, personal resources, political context, geographic location, etc. Rather, the objective is to introduce the cancer patient to the opportunities in *My Chronic Cancer*™ and in *My Cancer Advocacy*™ so that they become second nature.

After all, as cancer patients we are both the hosts and the customers. We are the ones paying the bills.

****

WIFM

What is WIFM? What does WIFM have to do with cancer?

At the end of each chapter is WIFM - "What's In-it For Me". WIFM is a reality assessment of what just happened, a take-away snapshot, a look-back perspective. WIFM is an opportunity for reflection, as: Should he have done that?, Would I do that?

WIFM is a way for us to question and measure our own goals and advocacy development against those of Ping, Pong and Penn.

WIFM introduces us to the *DNA-like Framework*™ concept, where *My Chronic Cancer*™ and *My Cancer Advocacy*™ are the twin strands of the *DNA-like Framework*™ that are connected by Base Pairs. Think of this structure as a ladder where the Base Pairs are the steps connecting the ladder's sides (the twin strands).

"Base Pairs" are our incremental achievements against cancer. So at the end of each WIFM is an assessment of how many "Base Pairs" each cancer patient built - Ping, Pong and Penn - likewise you. In the *BP Score Card*™ at the end of each chapter's WIFM we tally our "Base Pairs" for that chapter as the "steps" that link the twin strands of the *DNA-like Framework*™.

This is Not Cheating

With confidence and a methodology - It can be done.

Go ahead, look at Table 2 (Page 240) at the back of the book to see how Ping, Pong and Penn built – or did not build - their own *DNA-like Frameworks and Base Pairs* in each chapter of their cancer journey.

After all, I've already used this methodology to save my own life. So this book is about the same methodology for you to save your life in cancer, too.

Then, read the chapters – slowly - to see how to make the *My Chronic Cancer Advocacy* methodology work for you.

Dedications

No man is an island.

Arriving at Yale Cancer Center, I was out of chips. As I emerged from my fourth relapse I was down to less than three weeks of remission – likely none if I am totally honest. My immune system had been beaten-up and my cancer had learned to quickly and easily dispatch every new treatment I sent its way.

I had already met a lot of people like me with cancer. As we attack our cancers we destroy our insides, too, as we run out of options and out of time. While I had learned how to become my own advocate, I still needed competent medical help.

With sincerest gratitude this book is dedicated to the following three people, because without them I would not be alive to share this story and methodology with you.

• Dr. Francine Foss.

• Dr. John Murphy.

• Phyllis Bradley, my friend and cancer comrade. Against all of my protests my primary nurse struggled to convince me of the necessity of having a port implanted to receive my treatments. Then, undaunted, my nurse drafted Phyllis into her "Port Campaign". Over all my best defenses what my nurse had struggled to accomplish, Phyllis achieved solo with aplomb. I soon had a port! Yet, even as a true Type-A, Phyllis lost her battle against two concurrent blood cancers.

My respect for Dr. Foss, Dr. Murphy and Phyllis is without bounds. There is no possible way I could have prevailed against my cancer adversary without them. Relentlessly they cleared the path ahead. My sincerest hope is that you will be so fortunate to have a team and friends as dedicated, as competent and as caring as mine.

Table of Contents

Unintended Journeys in the Land of Cancer

Preface

June 2004: Two people who knew nothing of one another began to experience the onset of similar symptoms for two different cancers. Cancers that, unbeknownst to either of them, had been silently and progressively threatening their lives for decades.

Yet, not until May 2005 did they arrive at the same oncologist still seeking answers and help.

Still, they would not meet until September 2005 when she was in her sixth of thirteen chemo treatments and I was in my first of six CHOP treatments.

My friend, a pretty Italian nurse of thirty-three, had a curable cancer. She had had extensive medical training and had played by all the rules. But she is now dead. This is just plain wrong. I am unable to describe the deep pain I feel for the loss of my friend.

Me, I have an aggressive and incurable cancer. I have never had any medical training and I've always colored outside the lines. Yet, I am alive and have regained my health more than ten years past the onset of those symptoms for an incurable cancer that ruthlessly kills nearly all its hosts within just two years.

Why? Why? Why?

Far from posturing that I have all the answers, I wish to only offer that I hope I have some useful ideas to share with you.

While the daunting pain of the loss of my friend has become something I have been unable to move beyond, even in cancer I have learned some beautiful things about life.

I have learned that our best days are always ahead of us. That little kids and small dogs beat materialistic agendas every time. That life is irreplaceable. And, gradually, I am coming to understand that my friend's legacy to me is in seeing the real beauty of life.

Introduction

READ ME: Look at cancer this way – Cancer's only purpose is to kill and it does not take prisoners. Period!

So in cancer we are either on the offense, or we are on the defense. And in cancer we must always be on the offense.

In cancer if you are on the defense (1) you are behind and playing by cancer's rules, and (2) you are not wining.

To get on the offense against your cancer you will need goals, a plan and the means to achieve your goals. That is, you will need a strategy and tactics.

Start with these goals – in this order:
- 1st: I will live to be at least 100, and
- 2nd: I will reach a state of *My Chronic Cancer*.

Call it a "Mexican Standoff" if you want. Most important: you will not reach your 1st goal if you do not reach your 2nd goal.

Next, resolve to implement the tactics of *My Cancer Advocacy*, aka "means", to reach your 2nd goal. It will make your journey to your 1st goal easier and more likely.

Then, re-read again from the beginning until you get it. Period!

Cancer: My Cancer Never Sleeps!© is Part Two of *Putting the How Into Hope™* as the way to achieve *My Chronic Cancer™* as your strategy, by *My Cancer Advocacy™* as your tactics. What follows is a continuation of *Cancer: Who Gave Me Cancer?©* for you to reach goals #1 and #2.

Cancer: My Cancer Never Sleeps!© is about *Putting the How Into Hope* in the face of the show-stopping experience of being diagnosed as having cancer and about what comes next as we try

Cancer: My Cancer Never Sleeps!

to grab hold of our lives to address: What is going wrong?, What next? Where? and With who?

Through the continuing odysseys of three real people already diagnosed with cancer we are able to see ourselves to judge how we might respond. Would we be stoic, complacent, compliant, accepting but questioning, proud, assertive, fatalistic, irrational? Would we be pragmatic, pro-active advocates of our own cause, determined to prevail over our new adversary at any costs?

Probably, yes. But, then, hope fades as reality set in.

Cancer: My Cancer Never Sleeps! continues the vision of *Putting the How Into Hope.* This book is for all of us struggling with cancer and trying to make progress.

Cancer: My Cancer Never Sleeps! is not about faith healing, not about vitamin therapy or any vague alternative therapies. It's about integration of the cancer patient with his/her cancer resources and cancer technologies to prevail over our determined adversary. That is, it's about always being on the offense.

The proposition of *Cancer: My Cancer Never Sleeps!* continues the effective integration of the cancer patient into his/her treatment process as the third leg of the proverbial three legged stool.

The first leg is comprised of our "resources", like doctors, hospitals, laboratories, nurses, support teams, insurance and collateral providers like clergy, attorneys, etc... The second leg is comprised of "technology" that includes medications like chemos and biotech treatments, radiation, etc...

The third leg is us, the cancer patient. *Cancer: My Cancer Never Sleeps!* wants cancer patients around the world to see cancer two ways concurrently:

• First, cancer as a chronic disease. Once diagnosed as having cancer we have a life-long adversary we must confront every day for the rest of their lives. Yes, every day. Otherwise we risk conceding to cancer as our fait-accompli life-threat.

• Second, engage our cancer as our own advocates. As cancer patients we will make much more progress if we fully comprehend the life threat of cancer and apply it to develop our own cancer advocacy. Not as irrational ego, but with a positive offense and a long-term attitude against our cancer adversary.

Cancer: My Cancer Never Sleeps! strives to advance this integration by strengthening our awareness of cancer concurrent with development of *My Chronic Cancer Advocacy* with these attributes:

• Integration of the cancer patient as his/her own cancer advocate with the best available resources and technologies.

• Development of an adaptive plan-forward based on a positive attitude, while distancing ourselves from accusation, blaming, self-deception, denial and procrastination.

The means to achieve these goals are presented in *Cancer: My Cancer Never Sleeps!*. through three realistic role models: Ping, who is procrastinating, opinionated, left of center negative; Pong, who is moderately pragmatic, naïve, and right of center positive; and Penn, who is pro-active, insightful, analytical, decisive and selfish.

Although all three know one another, intentionally there is little intra-engagement so the book does not lose its way through the color of inter-relationships. Their individual wanderings in the land of cancer are essential to understanding cancer as a chronic condition and the necessity of developing our own *My Chronic Cancer Advocacy*.

Because cancer is a strong and determined adversary, it is not good enough to have the most advanced technology or the best resources if the cancer patient lacks the ability to see cancer as a chronic condition and fails to develop his/her own *My Chronic Cancer Advocacy.*

Cancer: My Cancer Never Sleeps! strives to *"Put the How Into Hope"* for all cancer patients by taking us on the journey with Ping, Pong and Penn. We see their real-life cancer experiences unfold and we see their "How" develop (or, not develop) so that the cancer patient truly becomes the third – supporting – leg of the three legged stool.

For the chapters ahead, here are a few pearls to help as guides:

• Ping's doctors' last names always begin with the letter "A", Pong's doctors' last names always begin with the letter "B" and Penn's doctors' last names always begin with the letter "C".

•   The journeys of Ping, Pong and Penn follow two concurrent story lines simultaneously. One is the individual personalization of cancer to our three patients as ordinary people, not unusual in any particular way. Second is the evolutionary nature of the cancer experience by each patient.

•   The book flows thematically so that each chapter is made up of five sub-chapters, one for each of our three cancer characters as they progress by stages through their own cancer challenges and "WIFM", as a reflective look-back at the end of each chapter and "BP Score Card to tally our successes.

•   In Chapter 1 all three appear again as veterans of their respective cancer treatments. By Chapter 4 we experience the stresses of cancer with each of them. By Chapter 7 each patient is forced to confront the cyclical nature of their cancer. Then, in Chapter 11 we are faced with cancer's end game.   We travel the same road as they travel in predicaments they never anticipated. Because, really, they are us.

• To avoid undue complexity the focus is on the progress of the individual through cancer, i.e. Ping, Pong and Penn and their cancer experiences. It is not the purpose of *Cancer: My Cancer Never Sleeps!* to disparage any treatment, protocol or to engage in extended rants against doctors or other providers.

• If there is a tendency on the part of the reader to see *Cancer: My Cancer Never Sleeps!* as the means to be critical of doctors or other providers, please do not do that. While those things happen, they are contrary to the purpose of *Cancer: My Cancer Never Sleeps!*

• Instead, please see a character's lapses as momentary expressions of their humanness and their limited information availability colliding head-on with their accumulated emotions. Keep in mind that in cancer "stuff happens". The goal is to maintain a positive attitude so as to continue making progress to defeat our cancer.

Cancer: My Cancer Never Sleeps! seeks to encourage a positive attitude and the ability to make progress in the face of extreme adversity.

We need to always be on the offense against our cancers. Always.

So in the words of Winston Churchill,
"Never, *Never, Never Give-up.*"

Welcome . . .

Cancer: My Cancer Never Sleeps!

Prologue

Nothing will come of nothing.

All three have been living with cancer for a few years, about three. In that time they've adapted their ways to the realities of how cancer moves-in to dominate our daily lives. Penn adapted, too, but differently from either Ping or Pong.

"Café Soleil" had become their meeting place with a table on the terrace overlooking the town park. Today was another of those get together updates. This time Pong noticed a subtle change in how Penn approached the steps to the terrace that overlooked the park.

It was the expression on his face that gave away that something was different.

"Hi, it's been a while since our last luncheon. Gee, both of you are looking great," Penn said as he arrived at their table.

Pong inquired, "I noticed you took your time crossing the park. You seemed captivated by the attractive lady on the other side. Someone you know?"

Next Ping said, "I noticed that, too. Please fill us in."

"I guess I can't hide anything from you two. Actually, she looked so much like my new nurse I thought she may have the day off. Totally caught me off-guard. But wasn't her," Penn, replied,

Not willing to let such a provocative opening pass, Ping chose to pursue the nurse-thing, "So, you have a new and pretty nurse. How do you rate such a benefits package?"

"Well, like everything else in life, there are two sides to the story. The first part is that for the past few months I'd been in a clinical trial program at a large cancer-centric hospital. At first the trial chemo seemed to be working and we thought the tumors were shrinking. Then, at the mid-point the whole situation began to reverse course and the chemo clearly was not having any success against the cancer. The tumors began to grow again, but more aggressively.

It was very disheartening, but I knew I had to keep moving. I went into the clinical program knowing the risks, but also knowing I needed something like a clinical trial to buy me time, even if it didn't kill my cancer. Which it didn't," Penn said.

Ping interrupted, "So you suspected from the outset it may not work, but you went ahead anyway?"

"Yes, you're right. I had been maintaining a list of treatment options and a list of oncologists. I compared oncologists who had direct experience with my NHL sub-type and the chemo treatments often prescribed and clinical trials. I did this by creating a simple spreadsheet of oncologists, hospitals, chemos and clinical trials. Seems complicated, but it was actually quite easy.

When it was clear the clinical trial was failing I had to find a replacement fast and the spreadsheet was the best resource. It showed there was an incredible match of an oncologist, of chemos, another clinical trial and a cancer hospital almost in my back yard. And I would never have known it without the spreadsheet. Easy. Should have done it back at the beginning," Penn replied.

"In your back yard?" Pong asked.

"Right, so to speak, and I didn't realize it. Anyway, I've just started into a new treatment program and it comes with a very pretty lady who is my primary nurse. Cancer is ugly, but I have a pretty nurse with a great accent. So each time I look forward to my new treatments," Penn said.

"Now I really am envious," Ping said.

But Pong was curious, "Was the clinical trial a bad experience?"

"No, not at all. It's just that the P3 chemo was ineffective against my NHL cancer sub-type. It may have worked for some other cancer, but it did not work for mine. In truth, I learned a lot and one of the most important things I learned was how to use a clinical trial more effectively.

As a result of that clinical trial experience, I've re-ordered my list of treatment options so that I now have a select list of chemos already approved for my NHL sub-type. They are now my priority go-to's. They are backed-up by a short list of clinical trials. And if all else fails a stem cell transplant." Penn said.

Pong interrupted, "And you said this was easy?"

"Easier than I would have thought at the outset. Because clinical trials are emerging events, I want to stay current on when and where they are available. But they come and go, so what is interesting today may not be open or available in the future. Likewise, a more attractive clinical trial may open-up so I want my clinical trials go-to list to be as current as possible," Penn said.

I asked my oncologist about clinical trials for my bladder cancer, but he wasn't keen to look into them at the time," Ping added.

"I had a similar experience with my oncologist for the melanoma," Pong added.

"My journey in the land of clinical trials was much more like feeling my way by Braille after I found that my specialist-oncologist was not solving my cancer problem. I suppose I could be critical of the clinical trial experience for some aspect of it, but overall it bought me the time I would not have otherwise had. And it helped me to better develop my cancer advocacy.

All-in-all it was a positive experience and I benefitted greatly. Sometimes when an experience fails to meet our expectations we disparage it to our own disadvantage. Clearly the *"P3 Clinical"* did not work for me, but a future clinical could be my best option at another time.

This experience has clearly enabled me to understand the proper roles of clinical trials and to prioritize them for my future treatments. I am much better prepared or the future," Penn said.

"Well, both Pong and I are doing fine in our current treatment plans, so I guess we don't need to go down the clinical trials road for now," Ping concluded.

****

But we're getting too far ahead . . .

Let's meet-up with all three - again - as they move into the build-out phase of their cancer challenges and find out what Ping means by "... for now".

Unintended Journeys in the Land of Cancer

Part II

Cancer: My Cancer Never Sleeps!

#1 The New-New Beginning

Delays have dangerous ends.

Ping: Ping has been in a second round of chemo treatment, this time with Cisplatin for his relapsed bladder cancer. As we catch up with Ping he is just completing his last Cisplatin treatment.

Cisplatin is a chemotherapy drug based on platinum which has been a mainstay in cancer chemo treatments since the 1970's. As a chemo veteran it has reached wide spread prescription in various cancer treatments – the good news. However, it has been eclipsed by much newer cancer treatment technologies and it can cause some very unpleasant adverse effects – the bad news. Against such conflicts a cancer patient who is practicing *My Chronic Cancer Advocacy* should be expected to ask "Why are we doing this?" But Ping did not.

Ping has not had a free-ride with the Cisplatin treatments, but he accepted them as part of the drill. Near the mid-point of the Cisplatin treatment program he began to develop neuropathy in his fingers and toes. It was mild at first, but by the end of the treatments the neuropathy had become painful, more durable and problematic.

Ping brought this problem to Dr. Allen's attention, but Dr. Allen argued that the focus should remain on killing the bladder cancer and there may be some collateral costs to achieve that goal. In the end Ping made a Faustian bargain: the neuropathy became permanent in his toes and advanced to real pain under his arches, making walks and standing for long periods of time uncomfortable. It also became a transient experience in his fingers. But the real question was whether the Cisplatin was killing the bladder cancer?

In other respects these Cisplatin chemo treatments had been nearly identical to the first round. Same hospital, local and easy to access. Same team, friendly and no changes.

"Thanks, hope this does it and I don't need to come back again. I have a follow-up appointment with Dr. Allen in a couple of weeks," Ping said to his primary nurse as he finished his last chemo treatment of Cisplatin. Walking out through the hospital's lobby Ping looked around and thought, "With all this in my backyard, why would I go to all the effort to go to a far-off hospital for such expensive doctors? Gotta-be nuts."

Driving home from the hospital Ping continued his logically ill-logical thinking, "Besides, all that clinical trials stuff is so over blown. Why go-off on some goop that's untried? Dr. Allen has it right."

The only remaining step before the next OV with Dr. Allen was the post-chemo CT scan. Same movie, as the saying goes.

By the time of the follow-up appointment with Dr. Allen Ping had already moved-on. The second round of chemo treatments had been so-so tolerable. And, as the post-treatment period faded into memory, he began to foster a sense of complacency. With Ping the way to avoid negative feelings was to make the leap to complacency. Just don't bother with the details. No euphoria, but a feeling of OK-ness based on nothing resembling rational facts. That's OK, right?

In the follow-up office visit with Dr. Allen they reviewed the CT scan as the definitive balance sheet on the effectiveness of the Cisplatin chemo against the bladder cancer.

Dr. Allen began first, "Well, Ping, I've read the radiologist's report and looked at the CT scan. From both perspectives we are seeing a definite shrinkage in the size of the bladder cancer versus before the most current round of chemo treatments. And from the scan we are seeing no appearance of any metastatic activity. While I do not want to say you are cancer free, I can tell you that we have not been able to locate any cancer in you. This has to be good news for you. Have you experienced any changes, like increased urination?"

"The neuropathy has definitely become more permanent in my toes especially, and frequently in my fingertips. If anything else, urination frequency has declined to a more normal level. But that's about all I've noticed," Ping said.

"Good. Then I think I should see you again in about 60 days, unless something changes," Dr. Allen said.

"OK. I am sure glad you steered me down the right road and away from one of those untried clinical trials. Let's hope this works."

"I understand. See you in couple of months," Dr. Allen concluded.

Pong: Being just on the other side of the net, the ball bounced differently for Pong than for Ping.

Pong was just then winding-up his second round of chemo treatments for the melanoma. "Really, was it just a simple relapse? Was it refractory? Why? Who's to know? Gotta move on," Pong concluded.

Anyway, this time their hope was that the Dacarbazine treatments and the surgical excision of the two remaining melanoma patches on his back would finally resolve the melanoma threat. But the ghost-like question was still there: if melanoma is supposed to be a manageable cancer - Right? - then, why was a second round of chemo and new surgery needed?

So much for "hope", Pong thought.

"Damn, this stuff can jam your head. Can't do my job. Can't even relate to friends and family like before. And I have no new data or info to backup why I am feeling this way. Something is driving these feelings that I can't reach. What is it?" were the thoughts in Pong's head, like a song on perpetual repeat no matter how much he tried to change the lyrics.

The chemo treatments and the surgery to remove the two patches had all been re-runs of the previous events – nothing new. Two weeks after the surgery and the end of the chemo treatments Pong returned to Dr. Black's office for a follow-up exam.

"This time your surgeries were larger than the first time and they are healing very nicely. But your white blood count is trending lower. That's new. From the outside you appear to have not had any adverse effects from the Dacarbazine treatments. How are you feeling?" Dr. Black asked as he checked Pong's vital signs.

"I've had some severe headaches this time and there was some diarrhea. I was a lot more tired during these treatments than in the first round of treatments with this chemo."

"Anything else?"

"Yes. I had a lot of nausea and came close to vomiting several times, but the anti-vomit medication seemed to work well and just in time. And I seem to have picked-up a dry cough. But I don't have a cold."

"Well, you are likely more intolerant of Dacarbazine now than you were in the first round. Its allergy season, so maybe you are just having a reaction. We'll watch you closely for other side-effects in our follow-up exams," Dr. Black said.

"Why? Is there concern over some headaches, the diarrhea and the white blood cell count?"

"With chemos like Dacarbazine we need to make sure there are no lasting effects, especially after a patient has had more than one round of treatment from the same chemo. Don't want to alarm you. Just being extra cautious. You appear to be fine.

Go out and enjoy your new life and I'll see you in a month." Dr. Black replied.

"Thanks. I'll try to do just that."

Penn: Unfortunately, Penn's situation was not as rosy as either Ping's or Pong's "appeared" to be. It was much worse.

Recall that Penn has a rare and aggressive sub-type of NHL, which is neither curable nor does it have a definite treatment regimen. Also, recall that he had been told by Dr. Childs, his first specialist-oncologist, to expect to live only about another two years, more or less, because his cancer was at Stage III when it was diagnosed and it had been diagnosed late.

So, by the time Penn entered treatment as a patient of Dr. Collins, he was in very bad condition and on track to validate Dr. Childs dire prediction. He would be dead in just a few months.

In fact, Penn's NHL was totally out of control and had been for at least six months, depending on one's assessment of the efficacy of the previous CsA and P3 clinicals. And the cancer was highly visible as enlarged tumors on the left side of Penn's neck, which also served to make him feel insecure and withdrawn. No matter what Penn did he could not escape the person he saw every time he looked in the mirror. He had nothing to celebrate and few reasons to smile.

Even arriving at the hospital for his new ZQT treatments was a struggle. There was the whole experience of dragging this cancer into another reception area, to another new cast of players, and another replay of the same shop-worn questions and forms to be filled-out, again. Then, the ultimate questions: Would it work? Where to next when it didn't work?

But there was the other side to consider. Mimi was supposedly a patient here, too. "Will our paths cross again?" he thought.

And, Dr. Collins had never said "No, you're beyond hope," but could have if he had been ....

"Penn, you've got a new oncologist who absolutely knows this disease. You've got the prettiest nurse on the planet. And they're taking you on with full-disclosure. Relax a little and get with the program. You can do this," were his thoughts as he arrived as a new patient, again.

"Hi. You're new here, aren't you? Glad you're here," the receptionist said as she caught him off-guard.

"Yes. I am a new patient of Dr. Collins and I am here for ..."

"You're Penn, right? I've already got your records here and I can get you started right away. Can you give me your birth date?"

Now, even more off-guard, Penn slowly mumbled the correct numeric sequence, like an automated tele-response.

"Good. That's you. Audrey will be out in a few minutes to get you started. She'll get your vital signs. She'll do the initial blood-draw and start you on the IV hydration. Then, she'll take you into the infusion area to meet your nurse. Let's see ... your nurse will be Sari, do you already know Sari?"

"Yes, I …" Penn started to say.

With the sincerest smile Penn had seen in a long time she said, "Good. Then, here's Audrey. Everything is going to work out just fine. Just relax. Sari's great. She'll take care of everything."

Audrey was a bundle of warmth and efficiency. She had mastered the art of making new patients in high states of stress transition to casual conversations about what their dogs and kids did last weekend, while simultaneously putting a needle in their arm and collecting their vital signs for the next hand-off. Essential, but hugely under appreciated.

Having learned all Penn's history of the past seven days, and gotten his blood draw and vital signs, too, Audrey had just dislodged Penn from the IV chair in her room and was walking him into the infusion room when Sari met them at the entrance to the same nurses' station where Penn had first been introduced to Sari by Dr. Collins. There she was, again, as pretty as the first time. "Penn, you're dreaming. Stop dreaming," he silently confided to himself.

"Hi, you decided to come back?" was Sari's opening line in that soft Mediterranean voice.

"Well, I figure this will keep me off the streets and out of the bars for a few hours."

"So are you saying you picked-up this problem in a bar? Hmmm. ZQT isn't intended to work on social infections. Or, could it be something more serious?" as she knowingly looked him eye-to-eye as his soft ping had just met her firm backhanding pong. In addition to being his pretty nurse, Sari had also mastered the art of being smart and tactfully quick witted.

"Let's have you sit in this IV chair. You've been through the IV process before, haven't you?"

"Yes, several times," Penn said, having wisely decided to avoid all clever remarks.

"OK. Then, this process will be identical each time you come in for a treatment, except that starting with your next treatment I will collect your vital signs and do the initial blood draw. Audrey gets new patients started and handles patients who will only be here once.

So I'll be meeting you at the reception desk from now on. Have you had any problems with chemo infusions in the past?"

"None." Penn said, having decided to just answer when spoken to.

"Good. But if the ZQT treatments are effective you could be receiving these treatments for a long time and you should start thinking about having a port installed to receive your ZQT infusions."

"Thanks Sari, but I'm just not interested in a port," Penn said defensively as Sari again looked at him eye-to-eye. No words were spoken, but she knew there was another agenda operating here and decided to let it lay where it fell, but not be forgotten.

"OK. Then, in cancer-speak ZQT is a non-chemo-chemo. You may have had lots of other chemo treatments, but I need to explain what to expect specifically with ZQT because these chemo protocols can be very different from one another.

First, after your blood-draw I'll start you on 500 ml of hydration and that will take at least an hour. During that time we will process your blood-draw to be sure your hematology and chemistries are within acceptable ranges. Dr. Collins will review the results and sign the order for your pre-meds and the ZQT IV, assuming all is OK.

We'll also start mixing the ZQT. And you'll start receiving your pre-meds. The ZQT IV will take one hour because that's per the ZQT protocol. Lastly, we will give you a second IV of hydration lasting about a half hour. So you should allow most of the day for a treatment. Sorry, there aren't any short-cuts.

Oh, yes, one more thing. Since this is your first day, Dr. Collins is in-clinic today and will stop-by during your treatment and we'll introduce you to our PA, Suzette. The three of us will be your primary contacts during your treatments.

And another thing, you'll soon see that I'm good at 'other things', if you need anything administrative in nature you should call Diane, Dr. Collins' AA. She manages Dr. Collins' schedule and is well organized. So are you ready for our personnel quiz?"

"No. I'm still back at the hydration-thing. Can that be with a glass of Sangiovese so we can avoid the pre-meds?"

"Were you planning on just making your cancer feel good, or killing it?", Sari said as she looked Penn eye-to-eye, again, while clearing the debris from the table after hooking-up Penn's IV treatment line.

"Damn. That eye contact and her soft accent, they're killers," Penn thought.

"Sorry. Just trying to make light of my problem," he said defensively.

"That's OK. I really do understand. I'm the one who should apologize. But what is Sangiovese? Actually, save that. Just got paged. I have to go to another patient. Don't forget about the Sangiovese-thing,"

After about half hour Sari returned with Dr. Collins and Suzette, the PA. As Sari attached the pre-meds to Penn's IV line and pump Dr. Collins introduced Suzette. "We're glad you were able to join us and we're optimistic about your treatments. This is Suzette and she will be my liaison in the clinic.

Because Sari is very busy each day with patients, you should direct your calls to Suzette if you need anything at any time other than when you are here for a treatment. We do this so our patients are never without access to us as a team. Before you leave today either Suzette or Sari will make sure you have a complete list of all our contact info.

Due of the aggressiveness of your cancer and the need to get you into treatment as soon as possible we did not schedule you for a PET-CT scan before today's first ZQT treatment. We still need that PET-CT scan, so Sari will have the scan schedule for you before you leave here today."

"Will that be a problem, that I did not have the PET-CT scan first?" Penn asked.

"No, because the PET-CT scan will be scheduled to take place very soon and the ZQT will not have altered the results. Besides, it does not matter. PET-CT scans are actually very precise balance sheets of the state of the cancer. We'll be doing several of these scans as you progress through the ZQT treatment process. It was more important to get you started into the ZQT treatments. Especially for our new patients, we need to know what is happening and when it happens. You already know how seriously we take each patient we accept, so please don't hesitate to update us if an unexplained event occurs or if an emergency arises. That's why we are here.

We've already discussed the ZQT chemo. It's a targeted therapy, so it will be quite different from your previous experiences. Also, don't expect too much too quickly. ZQT is targeted, but is can underwhelm those looking for quick results. We may have to get your system to adapt to it while it attacks your cancer. Both Suzette and Sari already have good experience with ZQT's side effects and can explain what to watch-for before you leave today.

Most important, don't be alarmed by the side effects. We've seen them all several times before and they are very manageable by comparison to your previous chemo experiences.

We'll start you at a high ZQT dosage level, but leave room to go higher if needed. I want to lower the activity level of your NHL cancer so we can see how the ZQT is performing. So Suzette will give you a prescription for a low dose of dexamethasone that I want you to take each day. You should also take a Benadryl at night, otherwise sleep will be nearly impossible.

While the dexamethasone will not kill the cancer, as a steroid it will slow it down. You should also take an antacid like famotidine about an hour before you take the dexamethasone. OK?"

"Yes, I can do that," was Penn's reply.

"Lastly, I really do understand your level of apprehension right now. I get it. I know how threatening these cancers feel in all of my patients. We are doing our best to bring your cancer under control. Just be confident in us and try to relax, as difficult as that may be.

We are totally committed to our patients prevailing over these cancers. Patients are not numbers to us. That's why we do careful evaluations and make dedicated assignments like Sari and Suzette. We all take an ownership in our patients. OK?"

Penn was then in disbelief and close to tears. Right now Dr. Collins could have performed a root-canal without Novocain and he would have said "OK. Sure. Please go-ahead". So, he said "Yes. OK. Sure," before realizing he had said anything at all.

Sitting in his new infusion chair Penn observed that patients came into the open infusion area, were treated and were on their way in what seemed like creative disorder, with nurses and technicians heading in all directions at once.

But Penn soon realized the activity wasn't confusion at all. It just seemed that way because here there were no walls of isolation. And, surprisingly, it quickly became obvious that the walls and barriers of the other hospitals where he had been a cancer patient actually prevented communication, thereby – unexpectedly - implementing confusion and inefficiency in place of innocently un-planned efficiency.

Penn had another interesting observation. Because the patients in this hospital were not isolated by physical or virtual barriers, they actually communicated with one another. Like in simple ways.

Even just making eye contact was a form of communication that often elicited a smile. On his first treatment day Penn saw how a simple "Hello" and some basic chitchat easily uplifted the facial expressions of other cancer patients. By comparison, none of this pro-positive experience occurred at the other more contemporary cancer hospitals where he had been a patient.

"Interesting surprise," Penn thought.

After the hydration and ZQT had completed Sari was back to detach the IV line, having completed the ZQT treatment and the last hydration in the sequence.

"Strange, this was different from my other chemo treatments. I expected some pain, some inflammation, something. I couldn't tell the ZQT IV from the hydration IV. I can do this," were Penn's upbeat comments to Sari as his first ZQT treatment was ending. Sari handed Penn the appointment with the radiology department for the PET-CT scan.

Then Sari began, "You'll probably experience some fluid retention in the first few treatments. That's normal and will go away. You may have some back pain and a headache. That's normal, too. It's OK to take some over the counter pain medication. Just keep it low and stop when the pain has gone away. If you get a lot of fluid build-up call us.

Here's our contact info [handing Penn the paper previously discussed by Dr. Collins and the dexamethasone prescription as signed by Suzette]. Just try to reach Suzette first. And remember, when you arrive next week I will meet you at the reception desk and we'll start you with the blood draw here in the infusion area.

And one last thing. I always give my new patients a hug at the end of their first treatment day [Sari gives Penn a sincere embrace]. Might fracture a few rules, but it's me. Besides, it's a custom in my family. We're glad you are here with us and I want my patients to know that I care about every one of them, like they are my family. You'll see.

Oh yes, the other thing. The Sangiovese...

Actually, hold-that. Just got another page. Tell me next time. Bye. See you next week," then, like Mimi, she was gone, too.

WIFM - Reality Assessment #1

One's delay is another's opportunity.

Ping: He is starting to experience the beginning of what the absence of cancer advocacy is likely to produce.   First, it produces mediocrity and antiquated solutions.

Then, in the long-run, it produces intractable problems. In the absence of his own cancer advocacy Ping got yesterday's cancer treatment.

Dr. Allen never looked into other, newer, treatment options. He never explored treatments with fewer or no adverse side effects? He never looked into targeted treatment therapies for Ping's bladder cancer.

But Ping dropped the ball here, too, because he never asked "Why is my oncologist prescribing this chemo against other less adverse, newer treatment regimens?   Nor did he ask, "At what collateral costs?" As we move forward we'll also explore other side effects and the consequence of secondary cancers.

Pong: His situation appears to be similar to Ping's, i.e. just another bounce of the same ball. But look closer. Pong's problem(s) are riskier.

He has just completed a second round of Dacarbazine treatments for the refractory melanoma. But this time he has experienced definite adverse effects he did not experience in the first round of Dacarbazine treatments.

Dr. Black said at the end of the office visit he would watch for indications of post-Dacarbazine treatment side-effects. But he left unanswered the lower trending WBC, white blood cell, count. This is not irrelevant. Where's the advocacy for his patient?

What if there is more to the adverse reactions in the second round of treatments than just routine side-effects? His mistake was to stop there. And he totally relied on the CT scan. He should have ordered a PET-CT scan to determine if the melanoma had spread beyond the two patches he had just removed.

After all, it's been several months since the first Dacarbazine treatments and this set of treatments and surgery were for melanoma that was refractory to the first round of treatments. Hello!

Penn: *If it was not a new-new beginning for either Ping or Pong, i.e. same old, same old, was it a new-new beginning for Penn?*

The answer is two-fold, both Yes and TBD. Regarding the "Yes" part, his new team and hospital know his NHL sub-type cancer, they take ownership, and the ZQT chemo - a non-chemo-chemo - is a targeted therapy. We can clearly see that his "My Chronic Cancer Advocacy" has taken Penn to places that Ping and Pong are not yet at.

While his cancer is a more threatening adversary than either Ping's or Pong's, several critical actions are now in process at the same time.

As for the TBD part, we can't know at this time because, as Dr. Collins said, "It will take a few weeks to accurately know how active the ZQT is against your cancer." But, unlike either Ping or Pong, it is true that Dr. Collins is an expert in Penn's NHL sub-type. And Dr. Collins is actively engaging the cancer through the dexamethasone to "... slow it down" to give the ZQT a chance to gain the upper hand.

Also, unlike either Ping or Pong, Penn's advocacy has placed him under the care of Dr. Collins, an expert in his cancer, inside a hospital dedicated to cancer treatments with a staff

that is fully integrated with the full range of cancer resources.

So, discount this if you choose, but Penn shows signs of actually having a new core team with the ability to get the job done. That is, to change certainty.

Lastly, of the three Net-Net assessments, it is a new-new beginning for Penn because his "My Chronic Cancer Advocacy" is now paying dividends to him.

<u>BP Score Card</u>:
Ping = 0, Pong = 0, Penn = 1 – From the initial diagnosis, but especially after the initial treatments, being at a cancer centric hospital with the right technologies, i.e. as two legs of your three legged stool, will be critical to the success of your long term offense against cancer

#2 Exercise, Diet & Other Health Points

Right. Some will and some won't!

Ping: On the surface nothing appeared out of the ordinary with Ping's daily habits. If anything they were as middle-class as they were possible to be. The only exception was the ever present neuropathy in his toes and lately his fingers. It was a physical reminder about cancer treatments that there were prices to be paid. No free lunches.

Unfortunately Ping did not connect, or did not want to connect, cause with effect. Beyond the bladder cancer other tell-tales were beginning to emerge, like gradually increasing blood-pressure above 140-90 and total cholesterol was now over 200. More specifically, his LDL and Triglycerides had been climbing for several years

But Ping was self-made, having risen from very modest beginnings with limited education. He and his wife had a comfortable, if not extravagant, life style and they liked to treat themselves to some of the trappings of their middle-class status.

Ping did not exercise on a regular basis because, he reasoned, a regular diet of physical labor was a concession to the exercise fad that had swept though the other employees where he worked. Often he would hear them talking, even boasting, about their 10K and 30K bike rides or their long jogs. To Ping there was enough exercise in his job and just getting the chores done around the house

There was the lawn to cut, must be a mile of walking there, the gutters to clean and always something to paint or the cars to wash. Even getting the place ready for a back-yard barbecue was no shortage of de-facto exercise. He knew that sitting still was not an option, so what was the "Big McGill" about so much exercise?

While he had smoked his share of cigarettes until recently, all the information of the past several years and the bladder cancer had convinced him to give-up cigarettes. But to give-up an occasional cigar and a bourbon or a beer was just over the top and too much to ask. After all, an occasional cigar with friends was like a rite of passage. And besides, an occasional cigar was nothing like a couple of packs of cigarettes a day. So, "Where's the harm?"

Just last weekend Ping and his wife had had a few friends over for a back-yard barbecue and Ping brought-up the subject of exercise and foods with a couple of the guys. Like it was already running as a background discussion anyway.

"We're having barbecued burgers and chicken. This OK with everyone?" Ping announced as a fait-accompli question from the grill on the deck at the back of the house. "By the way, Ed, you haven't become a health food nut have you?" Ping asked Ed and the group of men standing near the beer cooler on the deck.

"Not me. Don't buy into the stuff. Been doing just fine on the same food I was raised on. Don't see any reason to change. No problems yet," was Ed's reply.

"Good. Makes sense to me," Ping said as another friend nodded in agreement. "Besides, these health foods are for fanatics. They're fads that come and go. Just watch. This health food stuff is pricey and will die-off when people understand how much it costs," Ping said, while checking the burgers and chicken on the grill – some were already being blackened by the propane flames.

Pong: By comparison to Ping, Pong's cancer consequences had become more challenging.

First, the second round of Dacarbazine treatments had been what one might reasonably expect from a second round of the same chemo, with headaches and diarrhea that had not occurred in the first round of treatments. His WBC, white blood cell, count had been trending lower, too. Not too low yet, but there wasn't any definitive explanation for the steadily declining WBC counts.

Even if his cancer consequences were more challenging, Pong was doing better than Ping, at least when it came to exercise and food. This was mostly because Pong's pragmatism allowed him to be more attentive to his environment and to not have a knee-jerk rejection to new information.

Like others around him, in college Pong had smoked cigarettes, but largely as peer pressure in groups such as his fraternity. He moved away from cigarettes as the peer dynamic ebbed concurrent with the emergence of medical issues connecting cigarette smoke to lung cancer.

As he looked back on those experiences he found it pathetic that he had even allowed himself to smoke cigarettes at all. He knew they were bad, but he had allowed himself to get sucked-in. He realized that he got out of the pool when it wasn't the in-thing anymore. "Sure didn't need to follow that crowd," he often thought over the ensuing years.

He treated alcohol more pro-actively, mostly because he found the taste of hard alcohol mildly offensive versus either beer or wine. "Why drink something that doesn't taste good when there are very acceptable substitutes in beer and wine? And there are lots of really great tasting substitutes, too," was his line of reasoning.

"Interesting," he thought, "at Elaine and Jim's party last week there was no hard alcohol at all. No one asked and there was none around, anywhere. They were all good friends and no one had to have anything other than a beer or a glass of wine."

But if hard alcohol and cigarettes were out of favor, beef and chicken were still the preferred food choices. Pong had been raised on beef and chicken and it seemed that old preferences became habits that were not easily broken.

More important to Pong were trends, or more accurately, avoiding trends that were fickle and likely to cause a person to wander off the mainstream like smoking cigarettes had in college. To him such trends produced no visible benefit and some could actually do harm.

Just a few days ago Pong and a friend, Dave, were in a conversation about vitamins. Dave had asked Pong his thoughts on a new vitamin supplement he had heard of and was considering.

"I've never taken vitamins because I've always been healthy and I couldn't see how they would benefit me. Besides, the whole concept of daily vitamins seems to be faddish and to circumvent actively getting what we need from our regular meals," Pong replied to Dave about the new daily vitamin with an anti-cholesterol additive.

"Well, my cholesterol is borderline at 200. So I've been thinking of starting this new product because it could help lower my cholesterol while making sure I get all the vitamins I need on a daily basis," was Dave's logic.

"I see a couple of problems with that approach. First, maybe your doctor should be the one to make that decision. After all, isn't that why he is there for you anyway? Second, are you really sure the vitamin ad isn't just a promotional come-on to entice people? You look healthy and maybe your cholesterol level is not the problem you think it is. I would rather stay with my mainstream plan than begin to wander off the path just because I have been motivated by an ad based on unfounded fear. I have a plan and I believe in sticking to my plan. Maybe your problem is more that you don't have a plan and you're easily influenced by these promotions," Pong said in reply to Dave.

"I see your point about the idea of a plan. But I'm still going to look into that vitamin supplement. I like your idea. I'll discuss it with my doctor first," Dave said.

"Actually, my white blood cell count has been trending lower in recent blood tests, not by much, but lower still. I'm going to put it on the list of topics to cover with my doctor at our next office visit. This has been a good reminder. Thanks," Pong said as they parted.

Penn: Penn's situation was more challenging because his cancer was neither curable, nor did it have a specific treatment regimen. And before becoming a patient of Dr. Collins it had been out of control for the past several months.

Like Ping, Penn was experiencing a durable neuropathy mostly confined to his toes. It began at the end of the CHOP treatments and persisted on-and-off for over a year. It was Dr. Chase, his first oncologist, who had suggested he take a vitamin as a possible way to counteract the neuropathy.

At first Penn was reluctant to take the vitamin, thinking it was the equivalent of an old wives' tale. But when the neuropathy spread further into his feet and became painful in his arches he re-considered Dr. Chase's advice.

At times the neuropathy foot pain became so severe it made walking painful and over the counter pain medication was ineffective. He had no other choice but to try Dr. Chase's advice. And to his surprise it worked!

It wasn't durable, but it worked. Over time he found that he needed just one-half of the vitamin per day to control the neuropathy in his toes and the occasional neuropathy in his fingers. Even more importantly, it totally eliminated the inevitable pain in his arches and his heals.

Dr. Chase's advice about using a simple vitamin to forestall the neuropathy had other implications, too. The more Penn thought about how the vitamin had solved the neuropathy problem the more he realized he had been missing other opportunities to improve his overall health, especially in the context of his chronic cancer condition. "More of my own advocacy," Penn thought.

Although he had not been in contact with other cancer patients like Ping and Pong for a while, he had noticed several articles connecting foods with additives and health issues. He recalled reading articles about food additives, especially in red meats and about vegetables and fruits with other vitamins and about exercise.

As an avid reader he had read the articles, but hadn't really paid much attention. Now they all seemed to take on a new dimension that fit into the prospect of having more control over regaining his health. This would be especially valuable if Dr. Collins, Suzette and Sari were able to have success with the ZQT against his NHL cancer. "Why not give it a try? Might make their efforts more successful," he thought.

The more he looked into additives fed to animals, like cattle and pigs, the more dubious the proposition of those foods looked. In his reading Penn went from current news articles to intellectually informed writers dating back several decades, including several by Helen and Scott Nearing.

The Nearings had left metro-life in NYC and taken up subsistence farming in Vermont, and later in Maine. At the time they had argued persuasively against the killing and consuming of animals. "I can imagine their 'I told you so' response to the additives in our foods – not just meats – in contemporary society's food supply," he reflected.

Soon Penn had made a decision to begin transitioning away from red meats, and more specifically to a diet that would be permanently less than 10% red meats. Since he had never smoked in the past, he was glad to not have to fix that problem, too.

Penn resolved that his new diet would be more biased to seafood, vegetables, fruits and include a substantial increase in fluids. He reasoned that red meats offered little beyond an acquired taste, but seafood offered better nutrients, like Omega-3 acids, with reduced levels of cholesterol.

He also decided to totally eliminate blackened and smoked foods. The literature on blackened and smoked foods was strongly negative. And it had lots of consistent discussion linking their foods processing with several types of cancer.

"Why go-out looking to help my cancer breed at the same time as I'm trying to get rid of it? Maybe the best way to approach this idea of moving to a cleaner diet is to get some professional help," he realized.

At the next ZQT treatment Sari met him at the reception desk and took him directly into the treatment area. Soon he was tethered to the hydration through the IV line. After about a half hour a woman arrived at his chair and explained that she was the hospital's nutritionist for the blood cancers treatment area and was available to provide nutritional guidance to patient's during their chemo treatments. Her name was Charlene. But like in the Beatles song, everyone knew her as Charlie.

"I've done some reading about foods and fluids and I think it's time to give the whole subject of my nutrition some new thinking. Maybe this is the time to correct some past sins and to get onto a new track. What do you advise?" Penn asked her.

"We see it all. Every variation you can imagine. Most of the time when someone asks that question they're not as serious as they claim to be, so I'm not sure where to start with you. If you're really serious about getting onto a new nutrition program let's start with the basics and we'll see how far you go," Charlie said.

Clearly Charlie had become a veteran at ferreting-out fact from fiction and Penn knew he had to respect her. Besides being a nutritionist, Charlie was another of the resources available to all patients at this comprehensive cancer hospital. Penn knew he would be a fool to look any further.

"So let's take some basic steps and we'll see how you do. First, let's get your fluids in line. When you get up in the morning have an 8 oz. glass of water before you do anything else. Take a shower, shave or whatever, but wait 10 to 15 minutes.

Next, have a glass of juice with your breakfast. Keep breakfast simple. Next, at lunch have an 8 oz. glass of water in addition to whatever else you are having. Then, before 6 PM only have a 6 oz. glass of your choice. Might sound like a lot of fluids, but after you are into the routine you'll do it as though it's second nature. Are you still onboard with this plan?"

Penn nodded "Yes" as he made written notes.

"OK. Good. I'll make this next part brief. From now on you are totally off all smoked foods and there will be absolutely no blackened foods. I mean none, nada, zip. Nothing, OK?"

Again, Penn nodded "Yes" as he made more notes, then said "What's next?"

"Are you taking any non-prescription nutritional supplements or vitamins?"

"Yes, a multi-vitamin and another vitamin. The multi-vitamin is for trace elements that I may otherwise miss and the vitamin is for the neuropathy that emerged after the CHOP treatments. Both at the rate of one per day."

"Ok. But begin taking only one-half of each per day. [Visually assessing him] You're fairly lean and probably have a BMI, that's your body mass index, of 22 or 23, so you are probably taking about twice what you need anyway. People like you obviously make the vitamin manufactures very happy. Besides, reducing the daily intake by half will give you a margin to increase back to a full tablet if needed without compounding the daily dosage over-the-top," Charlie said with a veteran's exasperation.

"For now that's it. I've seen a lot of people like you who make big commitments then do nothing. So I've resolved to only pursue those who are truly serious. Prove to me you're serious and we'll keep making progress. Don't fix these basics and there's no point to doing a graduate course in nutritional health if the patient doesn't even do the homework. I've learned too many times-over that intimidation can be the best motivator. I'll see you when you come in for your treatments. I'll know whether you are pulling your weight," Charlie said with a wink.

"Oh, one more thing. I was looking at the results of your most recent blood tests and you are running a level of glucose, a blood sugar, that's a shade high. It's not terrible and I've seen a lot worse, but we ought to be thinking about it because it is just as important as the rest of your nutritional re-adjustment. Do you do regular exercise?"

Again, Penn had been caught flat-footed. First it was Dr. Collins, then Sari with her rhetorical quips. Now Charlie.

"Well, not as a regular exercise-like program, if that's what you mean. I am outside a lot and do a lot of physical labor around my home. Does that qualify?" Penn said hoping to get a pass on her question.

"Ahh, no. Doesn't make the grade. So I want you to add a ten minute walk to your routine each day. Keep your hands out of your pockets and just let them swing with your walking rhythm. Do that for the next four weeks and we'll re-check your blood sugar level. Ok?"

"Sure, but why?" Penn asked.

"Diabetes. For you it's totally preventative. Besides, the exercise is great cardiovascular, too," Charlie said.

"Damn, I came here for a chemo treatment and I've gotten an oil change and a re-alignment. Is this standard operating procedure for all cancer patients?"

"Yes, in a way it is. At this hospital we look at our patient's total health package. If we can get the cancer patient to fix a few obvious problems, like nutrition and exercise, we are likely to improve our own batting average by creating a healthier patient.

After all, you have a nasty cancer with lousy metrics. You came here because you're trying to regain your health. Trust me, a patient's advocacy gets noticed. We believe nutrition and exercise are essential parts of the total health package. Personally, I think it can make you happier, too. Think about it," Charlie added as she departed back to the nurses' station with a gentle pat to his left shoulder.

Charlie's challenge did get him thinking about the proposition, especially in a way he had not considered in the past. True, he had found ways to be his own advocate and that advocacy had brought him to Dr. Collins and to this cancer hospital. Against all the odds of surviving his NHL sub-type it was his own advocacy that had saved the day, or more accurately, had so far saved his life.

But Charlie's parting words implied something more. They meant that a communication channel had opened unbeknownst to him with the team at this cancer hospital about his willingness to go beyond the traditional patient standard. She meant that the team, surely Dr. Collins and Diane at first, had already evaluated Penn as a keeper.

"Cool, never saw it coming," Penn surmised.

Another two hours passed and Sari was back to detach the IV lines. With that pretty smile and a few words she placed a bandage over the IV insertion point on his arm and sent him on his way, like he was being sent home by his grade school teacher after a day of class, idiot mittens and all in place.

"Bye. See you soon," she said with a soft smile and a twist of her head, with her near back hair rolling like waves onto a beach. Then, like the waves slipping back into the sea she was gone.

Penn was still in a mild state of shock from the encounter with Charlie, and Sari's parting, when, as he left the infusion area and turned the corner to head down the hallway he could not believe what he saw.

There was Mimi. She had a smile and open arms that enveloped him in an affectionate hug and kiss. "I can't believe it. After all this time. What are you doing here?" were the only words Penn could muster.

"Let me see you [as Mimi stepped back with her hands outreached to his]. You look great. You're not here for a treatment, are you? What are you doing here? I've thought about you so much. Can't believe you're here," Mimi said in as much amazement.

Standing there in the middle of the hallway, oblivious to all others' comings and goings of other doctors, nurses and admin's, Mimi and Penn were locked in their emotional re-encounter.

"I've only been here a short time. Seems like I've traveled everywhere since those CHOP treatments. Lots of hospitals and lots of oncologists. I still have the same cancer, but now with very short remissions. Actually, looks can be very deceiving. It's been a very rough road this past year and a half. Even at home. But after all that has happened I'm less than surprised. Anyway, enough of me. What are you doing here?" Penn said with new excitement on re-encountering Mimi.

"I stayed with Dr. Chase, probably too long. I had a lot of problems from those ABVD chemo treatments. Gets ugly very fast. He was well meaning and very caring, but he just didn't have enough specialized experience and he wasn't associated with a major cancer hospital.

After those treatments I was doing fine for about ten months. Then, the same symptoms began to return, the itching and the red spots on my waist and back. It was even more aggressive than the first time. For the first couple of months I was very scared. Then I came here because I didn't know where else to turn.

Just before last Christmas I had an autologous stem cell transplant. So it's been about five months and I'm just now beginning to get back to my normal activities. I'm doing well, but ... [as Mimi glanced a look at the clock on the wall] ... I'm running late for my follow-up appointment. I want to hear about all your journeys and the home thing. Let's get together. Let's do dinner, or wine, or something. Call me," Mimi said as she reached out to embrace Penn again with another gentle kiss, then let go and moved away from him and down the hallway.

Standing there alone in the center of the hallway, half way between the infusion area with all their curious eyes and the exit doors, Penn was again full of all those old emotions. He had just been reunited with Mimi. Although she was gone again, she looked great. Mimi was really at this same cancer hospital and he would see his friend again.

Still in a daze Penn failed to notice that Sari had been watching the whole encounter from a distance, but had just moved to within a few steps of Penn when she said, "You two would make great movie material. A relative?"

"No. A friend. A very good friend. We went through our initial chemo treatments together. Mimi became my mentor. Unbelievable how much I've missed her.

"She's my patient, too," Sari said in a low consoling voice.

"Wow. I can't believe she's here. Just can't believe its true," Penn said, still dazed while looking down the hospital's empty hallway to where Mimi had disappeared.

"I'm going to walk you to the door so you can recover," Sari said as she gently put her right hand to the small of Penn's back and nudged him toward the reception area. "She's doing well, but she still has issues. Still a long way to go. I didn't know you two were so close."

Re-composing, Penn interrupted Sari, "A really great friend. Probably would not have made it to this point, but for her. I'm not sure if I'm making any sense."

"I understand more than you might think. For now let's just leave it there, OK? Remember, you have to be back here in a few days to explain that Sangiovese-thing. Don't forget," Sari said as she softly placed her hand on his shoulder, then let him go.

WIFM - Reality-Assessment #2

Without goals and advocacy,
human nature can be very resistant to change.

Ping. For Ping it is good there are only two ends of a candle to burn. It's not that he is a Type-A personality. Not Ping. It's that he is determined to live life his way with as few concessions as possible, even to recognized health threats. Especially those that conspire to worsen his bladder cancer. He had conceded the cigarettes, which he enjoyed, but had to admit that they were bad. But, sure-as-hell, he is not going to concede to the exercise fad.

Then there was the foods issue. Others could give-up on steaks and burgers, and get what in return? If cholesterol was the main concern, then just use leaner beef!

Clearly, Ping had learned how to rationalize any resolution he wants. He does not need a doctor to achieve that.

As this chapter ends, Ping has successfully rationalized the costs of healthier foods into a corner as being financial costs. His rationalization has eliminated the true costs to his health. Looks increasingly like he will be getting what he has been wishing for.

Pong. In a Ping-and-Pong match-up, Pong has been more open, more receptive to the impacts of exercise and food.

Unlike Ping, Pong learned two lessons about cigarettes: first, they are bad, no matter how they are looked at and, second, peer *pressure is not a legitimate rationale to engage in a bad habit. At least he said he learned the lesson of following the crowd. And with alcohol he had been an observer and decision maker.*

But, regarding foods, Pong had not yet mastered the trend away from protein foods loaded with dubious additives.

Returning to Ping, for Pong similar big health challenges are lurking ahead. His openness to discussion has alerted him to the small incremental decline he has noticed in recent WBC results. His sense of advocacy has motivated him to make a note to discuss the WBC change with his oncologist at their next OV.

***Penn.** While all three have cancer, Penn's blood cancer is a more aggressive life threat. And their paths continue to diverge, as we might have predicted near the end of "Cancer: Who Gave Me Cancer?"*

Penn is now in treatment at a comprehensive cancer hospital where the only patients are those with cancer. His medical team is totally devoted to his cancer treatment and to the treatment of other patients with cancer. And, unlike either Ping or Pong, his treatment progress is closely monitored by a dedicated team charged with returning the patient to good health.

Example, Charlie explained the cancer hospital's wellness philosophy and actually challenged Penn to pro-actively improve his health with specific exercise, food intake and control of supplements. That is, more engagement of Penn as the third leg of the three legged stool.

In contrast to Penn, with both Ping and Pong none of these health improvements are happening. And, given their medical environments, it's unlikely to go beyond casual conversations at best. Certainly not to pro-active challenges and regular monitoring.

Then, there is the re-encounter with Mimi, while Sari observes. Even these relationships are important because they are our new, real touch-point relationships in cancer.

Under such circumstances where would you rather be?

BP Score Card:
Ping = 0, Pong =1, Penn = 1 - Regaining your health in cancer means doing your part with the right foods, fluids and exercise. Get good advice, too.

#3 Inflection Points & Other Cancer Challenges

So he should have hated and feared Lion. Yet he did not.

Ping: At the outset, Ping just decided to ignore the re-emerging symptoms of his bladder cancer. Symptoms like increased urination with pain and dis-colored urine. He already knew these symptoms and had sub-consciously decided that if he ignored them they might soon go away. Besides, he was learning after having been treated with chemos for his bladder cancer to expect weird things to occur, sometimes at random.

He had long come to accept the neuropathy in his toes, and less frequently in his fingertips. Annoying as it was, the neuropathy did not seem to be on the same life threat scale as that imposed by the bladder cancer. Still, it was an annoyance and a quality of life issue.

It meant he felt cold faster when outside in the cold months. And it had become a durable reminder of the costs of cancer.

But, lately, there had been a slow increase in his urination frequency. This would not be so noticeable, except for the gradual increase in the accompanying pain. While it was not always present, neither did it permanently go away either. That was the nagging issue, it didn't go away. It didn't "resolve", as he had heard doctors describe problems that didn't exist anymore.

Was it related? Was it just part of a simple urinary infection that would eventually correct itself? Was it a holdover effect of the last Cisplatin chemo treatments? Was the bladder cancer making another threatening and undesirable return?

And the reverse occurred to him that he might be too anxious, too inclined to look for the worst. Still, it clearly overshadowed the neuropathy by a widening margin. "So," Ping reasoned, "is this

how it goes? What cancer doesn't accomplish with deadly tumors
in its host, it achieves by creating stresses that mount and mount
until the host dies of a heart attack or high blood pressure that
breaks vital plumbing. Damn, there's no answers and no end. OK,
I'll wait the four weeks until after Labor Day. If there's been no
improvement, I'll return to Dr. Allen."

Pong: As part of his regular follow-ups Pong returned to Dr. Black
at mid-summer. It had become routine for Pong to have his blood
work done ahead of the appointment and to discuss the results
during the exam.   This time Dr. Black had ordered a CBC
(complete blood count), a Hematology and General Blood
Chemistry tests. Otherwise the blood tests were no different
from his other blood tests of the past.

Dr. Black conducted a standard physical exam of Pong, carefully
examining his back to below his waist line, under his arms, his
chest and his thighs.

"If the ABCDE's are the standard guidelines for determining
whether a person has melanoma, I would have to give you a clean
bill of health. The excisional surgeries of the past have healed
well and I can find no other evidence of the melanoma. And all
your other signs and vitals look good. Just like they should," Dr.
Black said while looking down at the recent lab report of Pong's
blood tests.

"But," Pong said sensing there was more in Dr. Black's voice, like
he had not yet inserted a period at the end of his sentence.

"Even after you recovered from the chemos and the surgeries
your system stabilized nicely with your WBC in the 6.5 to 7.0
range. Yet, in the previous blood lab report your WBC had
dropped to 5.0. That's still above the lower end of the range at
4.0. But in this lab report it has dropped again to 3.8. Even your
other white cell values are not showing any signs of a problem.

Frankly, I'm puzzled because there are no other outward signs of a problem."

"Like, what kind of a problem?" Pong pressed on.

"Low white blood cell counts can be nothing if they recover in a relatively short span of time, like your body finally adjusting to all that it has been through lately. But a downward trending WBC can signal problems elsewhere."

"Could it mean there is more melanoma?" Pong asked, not yet willing to end the conversation.

"It could, but a low WBC is not a typical marker for melanoma. There can be lots of reasons for a declining WBC, but I'm concerned about the downward trend when your history has been stable at the mid-point of the range. We should look into this further. Let's have you do another blood test with more analysis. Then, we'll determine if additional tests or scans are needed. Stop at the same lab and have these tests done today [handing Pong the lab order].

The results will be back day after tomorrow. Make an appointment to come back that day," Dr. Black said, still studying the lab report for clues he had not yet located on the report.

After leaving Dr. Black's office Pong stopped at the lab as instructed and had the blood drawn for the tests. Another day went by, but Dr. Black phoned ahead of the appointment, "The lab report of your latest blood tests arrived and there is nothing out of the ordinary in the report, so there's no point in having you come into the office. I still want to solve this puzzle. Let's wait two weeks and have you return to the lab for another blood draw for the same set of tests. When I receive the lab report I'll call you to discuss, just like we are doing now. Put the date into your calendar. OK?"

"Yes, I can do that. I'll await your call," and Pong hung up the phone. Now, he was more bothered than puzzled. "Was this the harbinger of something more ominous?" he thought.

After two weeks and another blood test Dr. Black called again, "I have your lab report and all the results are within their ranges except for your white blood cell count. It has declined slightly to 3.6. You're certainly not in any imminent danger of infection, so not to worry. But I want to repeat this process one more time.

Same as the last. OK?" Dr. Black said.

"Sure," Pong said, now knowing that Dr. Black's voice had betrayed his efforts to hide the fact that he was pursuing an underlying idea.

After the latest set of two week blood draw sequences Dr. Black called again. "Your results are in and they are very similar to the last report. The white blood cell count is now at 3.5, slightly off from the last report. Let's have you come into the office tomorrow."

In the office visit Dr. Black conducted a brief exam of Pong and found nothing out of the ordinary. Even the previous melanoma surgery sites continued to heal well.

"Pong, on the surface nothing appears to be wrong and it would be easy to dismiss the declining white blood cell count because all of the other data points on the lab report are normal. But I think there is a message here that we need to pursue. After all these tests I am of the opinion there is nothing wrong with your white blood cells, but there's a problem elsewhere for which the declining WBC is the indicator, much like itching is an indicator of a problem elsewhere. Because of the previous malignancies I would rather err on the side of being safe, so I want you to have a PET-CT Scan next week."

"I've never had a PET-CT scan. What's involved?" Pong asked with a modest surprise.

"Very simple, [jokingly] you just lie very still for about 45 minutes. Actually there's a little more to it than that. Do not do any physical exercise for at least 24 hours before the scan and do not have any food for at least 8 hours before the scan. When you arrive a nurse will have you drink a contrast liquid and will inject a glucose tracer solution. You will lie very still on the scanner table as it is moved past the PET-CT camera. After you get on the scanner table it will take about 45 minutes. The PET scanner will record if a population of malignant cells up-take the glucose tracer.

After the scan is complete a radiologist will review the scan and file a detailed report. My office will receive a copy of the PET-CT report and I will call you to discuss the results. OK?"

"Do you think the melanoma is still active?" Pong asked.

"I'm not convinced one way or the other. I would rather assume the worst and be proven wrong earlier rather than later. That's why I believe we should do the PET-CT scan now rather than after another long sequence of tests. After the PET-CT scan report I am hoping to be able to continue looking for something less threatening. You still on board?"

"Yes, I am," Pong replied.

"Good. PET-CT scans are expensive. Upwards of $9,000 each. So I'll deal with your insurance carrier about the coverage. You'll only hear about it if I get a flat denial, but I've been here before. I'm confidant your carrier will approve the scan. Next, the hospital's radiology department will call to schedule the appointment. Just remember my advice about no physical exercise and no eating before the scan, else the scan can be worthless."

"Will do," Pong said with an uplift.

Next AM Pong received a call from the hospital's radiology department staff to schedule the PET-CT scan. The scan was able to be scheduled only two days out and the staff member reconfirmed what Dr. Black had advised about restricting both physical exercise and food intake. Pong was all set.

After arriving for the scan, Pong was given the contrast fluid to drink to make his digestive tract visible. Then, the technician prepped him with a glucose test to determine his glucose level, and the IV to inject the glucose fluid with the radioactive tracer.

While this part of the scan process made Pong apprehensive, the technician explained how the glucose would be taken-up by malignant cells and the tracer would show the location of the malignant cells to the PET-CT camera, thereby recording in 3D the exact location of any malignant cells in Pong's body. That is, if there were any there that were able to uptake the radioactive glucose.

"So, I'm Troy and the glucose with the radioactive buzz is the Trojan Horse. What have I signed-up for?" Pong thought apprehensively. The technician had obviously encountered lots of "Pongs" in the past and quickly assured him of the inherent safety in the entire PET-CT process. She even said, "When the scan is over I'll take you into the control room and show you your scan. It's what we call our Obi Wan demo. You'll see." All she left out was, "Trust me".

After about an hour of start-stop-start sliding through the PET-CT scanner's donut hole on the scanner's moving table the scan was over and the technician arrived to take Pong into the control room.

There, on the wide screen LCD monitor, was Pong in 3D, aka Pong as Obi Wan in hologram form. The technician explained that she was not allowed to interpret the scan image because only the radiologist had that authorization. On the screen she pointed out his internal organs that showed grey-black from the contrast fluid he had drunk soon after his arrival.

But when Pong asked about the two clusters of black dots that appeared like small pencil marks in his chest, the technician again said she was not allowed to interpret the images. However, she did offer that the black dots in PET-CT scans normally indicate the glucose tracer solution had been taken-up by malignant cells.

Emotionally rattled by what he had surmised from what he had just seen and heard, Pong did everything within his control to maintain his composure, thank the technician for the narrated tour and leave as quickly as he could. "No wonder the white blood cell count is headed south. The trick worked too well," he thought. "The Trojan Horse had just been welcomed into Troy. Damn!"

Next, was an office visit two days later with Dr. Black, Pong's oncologist.

Dr. Black had already reviewed the radiologist's report before Pong's arrival and had determined a discussion course based on the obviously adverse information in the PET-CT scan.

After the normal introductory pleasantries Pong asked, "I saw the initial images from the scan and from my limited information it looks like I still have a serious problem, right?"

"Your PET-CT scan clearly identified a few very small locations of possible malignant activity [as Dr. Black pointed to the PET-CT scan's black dots on his computer screen].

We could speculate, we could schedule you for a surgical biopsy or we could conclude from the scan and the radiologist's report that the activity is due to your experience with melanoma. I am of the opinion that the latter is the right conclusion. You've had two treatment plans with Dacarbazine, a standard of care treatment for melanoma.

In my opinion your cancer is refractory. That is, it's resistant to the chemo. And it has metastasized beyond the original sites we removed. Melanoma is quite capable of doing that.

Because your melanoma appears to be resistant to the Dacarbazine, I believe we should enroll you in a clinical program where you can receive more advanced treatment than would be available by opting for another round of Dacarbazine treatments. Are you with me so far?"

Pong was still emerging from his state of shock but able to reply, "I think so."

"OK, good. I've already begun a search of clinical trials in melanoma, especially those for which you would quickly qualify and those that would be reasonably close. I've identified three, one of which is close by at a major hospital and sponsored by a major biotech, it matches your situation well and I have met the oncologist who is heading the trial. I have already discussed your treatment history, without divulging your identity of course, and we agree that you could be enrolled in the trial."

But Pong had some concerns, "Are there no other standard treatments? Could the PET-CT have just identified some errant Oreo cookies? We had previously ruled-out a clinical trial, but now we're about to change course 180°. What are the risks?"

"All very good questions. Let me take them in a different order. I wish it could have hit on some Oreo cookies. I sincerely do. PET-CT is a fusion of two scans, the PET and the CT. Essentially the CT scan is an anatomical scan, using X-rays to generate a detailed scan of you anatomically. The PET scan provides scan related data based on the uptake of a radio tracer in glucose by cancer cells. When the two scans are fused we are able to see with very high accuracy the location of cancers that – with much regret – have nothing to do with Oreo cookies. So we are confident about the cancer and its locations.

Second, you're correct. There are other standard treatments available, but I am concerned that because your melanoma appears to be resistant to Dacarbazine it will likely be resistant to other such chemos as well. I think we need a more advanced treatment approach.

Third, yes, we did previously rule-out a clinical trial. But we did so at a time when you did not appear to have metastasized melanoma. The PET-CT scan shows that the situation has changed, as is too often the case with a disease like melanoma."

Pong's turn, "And, the risks?"

"I see two types of risks. Risk one would be to do nothing, like 'Watch and See'. In my opinion this option imposes an unacceptably high risk because metastasized melanoma is a high risk cancer.

Risk two relates to the clinical trial itself. In the US clinical trials are highly regulated and have well defined protocols, so you know in advance what is expected and what to expect. For the clinical trial at hand, for you we are looking at a trial that has already produced good data, it is in Clinical Stage III, meaning it already is showing good indications. I've intentionally stayed away from those in either Clinical I or Clinical II.

You will have an oncologist for the clinical trial and I will continue with you locally. No interruption. If I were in your shoes, I would go this route."

Pong knew the ball had just arrived back on his side of the table, "I hear you. You're right. Let's go forward with this plan. What do I do next and when do I start?"

"Good. Let's get started. You'll need to sign the consent forms with my secretary and she will make copies of your history to send to the hospital. You will be seeing Dr. Butts and his resident who will get you started ASAP."

"Sure wish we could be could have had a different conversation," Pong said as a last resort.

"I do, too, but the experience with melanoma is that the patient has to assume ownership for his cancer, just like you are doing now. Delays can be costly," Dr. Black said in reply.

Penn: Having just completed the PET-CT scan at his cancer hospital Penn already knew what to expect. There was a blink-test ahead of him and he knew it was going to be ugly. But he knew, too, that he had to know. More to the point, he knew he had not come this far to wuss-out now.

What the PET-CT scan revealed were several black dots clustered along the left side of his neck and throat. Small dots and clusters of small dots. But what the radiologist's report revealed was worse. In unforgiving medical-eze, it described at least eleven significant tumors spread out from his left sub-mandibular region down to his clavicle.

These eleven tumors were all, but one, in his lymph nodes and ranged from a couple the size of a pea – about 4 mm in diameter – to several larger tumors ranging up to 2 cm long x 1 cm wide. The one stand-out tumor was big. It was outwardly visible and just under his left jawbone at 3 cm long x 1.5 cm wide. But worse, this rogue was where a lymph node had been before the last biopsy. With this PET-CT scan and report there was no doubt about what was causing the pain. Nor was there any doubt about where the next nuclear war would be fought in him as ground zero!

What remained unclear was whether the ZQT non-chemo-chemo targeted therapy was capable of reaching and killing his NHL targets.

Quite literally everything hinged on whether Dr. Collins and the ZQT were capable of killing his aggressive cancer that had faced no serious counter-attack in about a year. Penn did not have to be reminded that these bastards were now battle hardened terrorists intent on nothing less than his destruction.

So just as Ping was rationalizing how to avoid going back to Dr. Allen about his resurgent bladder cancer symptoms for another four weeks, and as Pong was then completing his first PET-CT scan, Penn was entering his third treatment cycle with ZQT and emerging from his first PET-CT scan.

But it was different here from all the other hospitals and patient care teams Penn had experienced. He saw Dr. Collins at the start of every cycle and on an as-needed basis. Then there was Sari. Sari was just there all the time. At least that's how it seemed because this hospital and this team in particular had become his new center of gravity.

In other words, he was benefiting greatly by being their patient. He had to admit that he had been captured into their orbit of care.   And for once in a long, long time he was feeling hopeful.

The obvious threat was posed by the tumors in the PET-CT scan, but Penn had a real sense of hope about this team and this hospital that had never really existed over the entire course of all the previous treatment plans.   At least after the CHOP treatments, everywhere else there had always been the ever present agenda of "Where to next when this plan fails?", always the expectation that the current plan – whatever it was at the moment – was just one more stop-gap measure to make on the road to getting to the next treatment plan as-soon-as-possible. Always another ticket to punch.

One has to wonder when, even with the most ardent Type-A personality, when will one finally cave in to failure after failure as our bodies erode away with each successive – and failed - chemo plan? Sure, one could argue defiantly in favor of never giving-up. But when there's nothing left to work with, when the chemos have eroded away everything from the inside, how does one continue-on defiantly?

Penn was actually sensing how to not have to do that at this hospital. Through perseverance, call it "Advocacy", he had found in Dr. Collins an oncologist who understood his NHL sub-type cancer well and who was confidant at prevailing over the cancer. No one else had exuded such confidence. "This is one incredible team," Penn confided to himself.

Back in reality, Penn was well aware that it was one thing to feel good about your team, while it was another to actually kill the cancer without losing the cancer patient, too.

At the start of ZQT cycle #3 Penn and Dr. Collins met to review his status and the PET-CT scan radiologist's report.

Dr. Collins began, "We could say there is good news and there is bad news, but let's just look at your situation as this is where you are today, OK?"

"Sure," Penn responded cautiously.

"Good. Then looking at your lymph nodes today [as Dr. Collins gently examined Penn's lymph nodes in his neck and throat] I am of the opinion they are not worse than when you began the ZQT treatments. I can't tell if they have shrunk very much, but I am certain they have not grown in size or gone beyond Stage II either. That's important for advanced stage patients with this NHL sub-type because ZQT can be underwhelming when they're looking for signs of improvement.

Also, you seem to be tolerating the ZQT treatments well. So I guess we could look at both of those as good news. On the other hand the PET-CT scan report has revealed some large masses here on the left side of your neck and under your jawbone. We just may have to be prepared to deal with these tumors separately down the road.

But I believe we should see if the ZQT can do the job first, before we take separate action. The fact that we are not seeing more tumor masses below the clavicle seems to indicate the ZQT is actually being active against your cancer."

Penn saw the opportunity to question Dr. Collins' pragmatism with, "But shouldn't the tumors have begun to shrink by now?"

"Sorry to personalize it, but your cancer was allowed to grow un-challenged for more than a year. One of the mistakes often made in treating patients with cancer is to jump from one treatment plan to another when we do not see instant results. Your cancer is well entrenched – much like hardened terrorists – but in the ZQT treatments we are not seeing the cancer advance beyond when you arrived here.

If the ZQT were not being active against the cancer by this time in the ZQT regimen, I would have expected to see it along your chest and under your arms. But the PET-CT report clearly shows it's not there. It has not been able to advance. So, for several reasons, I feel positive about continuing with ZQT just as we are. Patience and vigilance are rare but essential virtues in the treatment of these aggressive cancers," Dr. Collins replied with a definite hint of confidence.

In resignation Penn decided to retreat so he just said, "OK, I think I see."

Dr. Collins sensed Penn's doubt, but was not yet finished. "That does not mean we will not adjust our plan to meet the situation. We may need to do that and we have other tools available. But we need the ZQT and the cancer to show us the road ahead. Which they will.

And, this is very important, you must understand that you have stopped burning time. You are now in a place with an entire team dedicated to solving your cancer problem and to saving your life.

You fought hard to get here, and you should be very pleased of that accomplishment. Your advocacy won that day. You really did it. But now you need to back off and let your team manage your future treatments. I know how hard it can be for people who have fought so hard, for so long against such daunting odds to let go, but please let us do the job you have asked us to do.

I am truly sorry about your previous treatment history and I know how much you would like to be free of this threat. But we now have a solid baseline with ZQT and the PET-CT scan. With only three treatment cycles completed we appear to be seeing

ZQT be active against the cancer. This is very good news. You need to stay the course."

Penn knew he had a solid advocate in Dr. Collins. He also could see it was time to tack into fairer winds. This time he responded with a smile and much more up-beat, "OK, I get it. I'm on board."

"Good. Then, let's find Sari to get you started on your treatment."

WIFM - Reality-Assessment #3

Because, like Lion, cancer was to change all life going forward.

Ping. *In cancer, denial can come easily to some people. After all, in cancer it is often hard to see your glass as being more than half full. But denial is never a rational strategy in cancer. Ping is veering away from staying close to his oncologist. This is especially important at the earliest indications of a failing remission when it may still be possible to restrain the cancer.*

Re-examining Ping's thinking we find that he has no strategy, no deterministic tactics, no end game. He has seen this movie before and he just does not want to see the same scenes again. Neither do any of us with cancer, but Ping is just making a difficult situation worse and riskier by not at least re-engaging with his oncologist at the earliest signs of a failing remission.

Pong: *Imagine what would likely happen if Pong had not had the PET-CT scan? Right! In metastasized melanoma Pong's life threat could increase exponentially because he would have no reliable benchmark. Is he headed in the right direction into the clinical trial?*

What we have learned so far is (1) when the diagnosis turns against you, get a second opinion ASAP, (2) make sure you are already at a comprehensive cancer hospital and (3) you already have a plan with options identified by doctors who specialize in your specific cancer and treatments - with the treatments divided into A's (available now) and B's (soon to be released, including clinical trials with pre-qualified accessibility).

So how does Pong fit our model? Answer: He misses it by miles. He is off on a flyer to a new oncologist with whom he has zero experience, into a clinical trial with no preparation other than that he can be admitted - sound familiar?, without the benefit of any second opinions.

Although he will be at a cancer hospital for the clinical trial, there is a big problem. He will not be at the cancer hospital as an actual patient of an oncologist whose practice is at the cancer hospital because he will only be there to participate in the clinical trial. He will not be there as a patient in regular treatment for his metastasized melanoma. The difference between these two paradigms is huge because he could fall through the cracks of mis-communication. At the rate at which metastatic melanoma can spread such a patient could quickly pay a huge price.

So the answer to the question is, "Not as he should, but keep your fingers crossed."

Penn: Before we ask a similar question about Penn, let's recap his situation. He is already at a comprehensive cancer hospital. His medical team has deep hands-on experience in his NHL sub-type with a specialist-oncologist, a nurse practionner, a primary oncology nurse and a back-up team of nurses.

He is now in treatment with a targeted therapy for his cancer and early indications are that it appears to be active against his cancer in an environment where he is closely monitored. In brief, Penn would find it very difficult to be in a more favorable setting.

Against Penn's setting Ping is flying solo. He has elected to defer re-engaging with his single practionner oncologist for the next several weeks, even though he has acknowledged the likely onset of the return of his bladder cancer symptoms. In response to the ball that landed in Ping's court, he has turned his back and walked away in denial. To be sure, his cancer is not likely to cut him any slack just because he is in denial. **Cancer does not make such deals.**

Pong is much like Penn in that they both have just received PET-CT scan reports. But Pong has none of the supportive infrastructure of Penn. Instead of referring Pong into a comparable cancer care environment similar to Penn's, Pong's oncologist opted to roll the dice on a clinical trial with a new oncologist with whom neither Dr. Black nor Pong have any experience. **In a setting of metastatic melanoma this could be akin to playing Russian roulette with your life.**

Again, Penn went through a much more difficult course to this point. He has a cancer that is as risky as Pong's, but he is receiving a much higher quality of care because he has already learned the value of his "My Chronic Cancer Advocacy".

That being said, Penn is not without a difficult challenge.

As the chapter closes a new question has evolved, as put forward by Dr. Collins in, "But now you need to back-off and let your team manage your future treatments. I know how hard it can be for people who have fought so hard, for so long and against such daunting odds to let go, but please let us do the job you have asked us to do."

This is a very big issue on which Penn is being asked to leverage everything he has worked so hard to achieve. Will his cancer advocacy morph into him becoming a team player? Does he really have confidence in his team? Can he make that transition in the face of the news from the PET-CT scan report? Would you?

BP Score Card:
Ping = 0, Pong = 1, Penn = 3 – You must stay engaged as your own
My Chronic Cancer Advocate.
– Inflection points are critical. Do not let the process get away from you at any cost.
– Be prepared to evaluate your team and to accept/reject your team.

#4 Life's Stresses in Cancer-time

So, would you stand-up and walk out on me?

Ping: One of the problems with cancer, any cancer, is how it arrogantly adds new and complicated stresses to our lives. In effect it says, "Whatever was important to you is no longer important. Your cancer has usurped the critical path in your life."

Ping was not one to deal with new stresses well. If the new stress was something beyond his skillset, he deferred, procrastinated, ignored, enjoined, sometimes even denied its existence. He otherwise avoided facing the problem. This even seemed to work, sometimes. Like, when his phone system at work failed.

Sure, others complained about not being able to reach him, but at the end of the day someone else at work would get the phone fixed. Unfortunately this approach can become a crutch that too easily becomes a pattern in our future.

But cancer is unlike a dysfunctional phone system. And Ping's avoidance did not work with cancer because cancer has its own agenda, i.e. its host's eventual destruction. Deferral and denial just beget the end result we do not want, but with certainty.

Ping had already rationalized delaying a return to his oncologist about the re-occurring bladder cancer symptoms. But not returning to Dr. Allen did not impede the cancer or bestow any benefit on Ping. Instead, the cancer just went happily about its business unimpeded.

Running background, so to speak, was the accumulating burden of Ping's internalized stress build-up.

At home, over dinner, his wife asked, "Any further thoughts about returning to see Dr. Allen?"

"So far the symptoms have been manageable. Nothing more than a small increase in frequency and the pain level has been very low," was his reply while he busied himself heads-down with dishes at the sink.

"But shouldn't you make sure it's not returning, or returning faster this time?"

"I think I can handle it at this level," Ping said with a new hint of defense.

But his wife had a point she had not yet made, "I understand and maybe I would feel the same way. You've been at this for a long time now and we've seen this problem twice before and it always seems to start the same way. Like with the symptoms you've been describing. Is it possible? I mean you could get another opinion, like from a specialist?"

"Do you not have confidence in Dr. Allen?" Ping was quick to reply.

"Sure, I have confidence in him. He's always responsive and he seems to have a good level of understanding of your cancer. But wouldn't you feel more comfortable with a second opinion, even if it just re-confirmed what Dr. Allen has been telling you?" she said with more directness now that she was getting to her point.

Ping was feeling more defensive about deferring his return to Dr. Allen and about seeking a second opinion, like with a sense of having been backed into a corner.

"I've been with Dr. Allen now for more than three years. Even with a nasty cancer like mine, he has stood by me all the way. How do I know someone else would do the same? How do I know someone new would be as experienced with my history and my cancer as Dr. Allen? How do I know that going to another oncologist wouldn't end-up being taken as an insult by Dr. Allen?

Could happen, you know. I am holding-off returning to Dr. Allen until – and because it may only be an infection and not the cancer – until it has become as much of a problem as in the past. And it hasn't reached that level yet."

His wife was not yet ready to give-up, "Ok, all that makes sense, but aren't you actually hurting yourself by holding back until, as you say, it has become as much of a problem as in the past, because don't we already know that the cancer gets worse? I mean, it gets stronger each time it returns. So aren't you increasing the risk to yourself by delaying a return to Dr. Allen or in getting a second opinion? "

Doing what we all do when the pressure gets to be too much or when our own arguments are obviously beginning to fail, Ping replied with a hint of anger at having been pressed beyond his comfort zone.

"I would like to find-out if I just have a simple infection and not jump at every hiccup to return to Dr. Allen and have him put me on another chemo because … I mean … just to be more safe than sorry. Can we just leave it there?"

"OK. Sure. But you're sounding like a tourist, like you might do this or might do that. Your cancer, if that is what it is this time, is a real life threat. I just thought there might be a couple of different ways to look at these symptoms this time." she said in quiet resignation.

"Damn-it. You just won't let me have the space I need. How can you know my situation better than me? How can that be?", Ping exploded, raising his voice and looking at his wife face-to-face.

Raising her soft voice too, "Ping, that's just not true. I'm more than a spectator here and I believe I am seeing the same symptoms for the third time, but with the experience of having seen them twice before. How can you expect me to stand here and not speak my mind, especially when I honestly think you may be making a big mistake?" she said having made point.

Looking away from her while hanging the dish towel on the handle of the oven, Ping realized he had no cards left to play. Down deep he knew very well where her loyalties lay.

Taking a deep breath he replied, "OK. Let's do this: I'll give this plan of mine two more weeks, till two weeks from Monday. If there's been no improvement, I'll call Dr. Allen for a new appointment. I'm still not keen on the second opinion-thing. But if there's been no improvement in the symptoms by then, I will call Dr. Allen for the appointment. OK?"

"OK, sounds like a plan," she said as she closed the distance between them to give Ping a hug and a gentle kiss.

Pong: Pong was feeling fine. Outwardly there were no adverse signs, no visible symptoms. Nothing appeared to be amiss. But the real story was unfolding locally unabated, just out of view.

Sub-consciously Pong felt discomforted by the tension of the recent PET-CT scan and report that pinpointed the melanoma enclaves evolving within him where his vital organs lay within easy reach. All this was conflicted by the outward appearance of a healthy person who appeared to have beaten one of cancer's most deadly adversaries.

Just a couple of days after having seen Dr. Black Pong was conversing with a few friends at work who had known of his cancer experience and who congratulated him on winning his bout with the melanoma. Pong did not want to introduce a sudden scare to them with the recent PET-CT news, so he was casual in accepting the praise. He used the moment to suggest that he would still need more time to have a solid level of confidence of success. Still, he was not able to allow that cancer could become a chronic condition. Nor did he see a role for his own advocacy. Too bad for him.

At the end of the work day Pong often sought release from the tensions he experienced in his job, and from the cancer, on a bike ride with friends like Dave from the earlier discussion about the vitamin supplements. Today's ride had been brief, only about 10K out and less back as they took a shorter route on the return. Pong pulled off at a country general store for a water and granola bar. Dave did likewise. On the front porch of the store Dave began, "Beautiful ride, no matter how many times I've been over that course. I just love it. You seemed to be doing well on the hills, like all the internal machinery is ticking-along just fine."

Pong saw the opportunity, "Overall I'm doing fine, but once scared by cancer you're always looking over your shoulder. My doctor has me in for some more routine tests and scans. I sure wish the rear view mirror wasn't always in my line of sight."

"I guess I'm fortunate because I have no experience with anything like cancer. Not sure how I would react, either. Oops. Sorry. Didn't mean to touch on a tender subject," Dave said.

"That's Ok, not a problem. These rides with friends are a great release, more from the what-ifs than anything else. At least they keep my focus on other things, like the road ahead – not the one behind," Pong said.

"Sounds like you are all through with the treatments?" Dave inquired.

Looking across the road into vineyard and after another bite of his granola bar and some water Pong replied, "For now, but something could show-up on a test and I could need another round of treatments, even to enter a clinical trial. We have no way of knowing. And I pray it doesn't happen."

Dave had become curious, "Having been through some cancer treatments did you see others who became religious as they were going through their treatments?"

"Actually, that's an interesting question. Until I was half way through the first treatment plan I had not thought about religion relative to my cancer. When I did it seemed disingenuous to me because, while I have my religious beliefs, I am not a card-carrying church-goer. There were moments when I felt fear and when I questioned how I might address the religious issue, but I felt uncomfortable about becoming someone I had not been in the past.

The more I thought about a religious dogma the more I felt like I would be switching sides at the last minute for all the wrong reasons. While I felt the fear, I did not want to become phony just due to the cancer.

One of my thoughts was, 'If I became a born-again something how would I feel if I recovered?' It was a very uncomfortable proposition, maybe even an added a different incentive to regain my health.

My wife goes to church now and then, though not on a regular basis, and she has a more defined religious road-map. Through both treatment plans she didn't press her religious ideas on me, but I knew they were there all along. She was a solid rock by my side all the time. Hadn't thought much about it till now, but her religious roots probably helped make her stronger than me. Still, I felt uncomfortable switching horses in mid-stream because I was having a tough go."

Looking to move on Dave said, "What's next, or are you all through for now?"

"My doctor wants to keep our options open, so he's looking at things like clinical trials in case something flares-up down the road. But for the time being everything seems stable," Pong said to bring an end to Dave's questions about the treatments?"

"That's great. Congratulations on the accomplishment. Say, it's getting late. I'm going to head home. I'll see you tomorrow."

"Have a safe ride home. See you tomorrow," Pong replied as he also got back on his bike for the short ride to his house.

Penn: "Dinner," Penn's wife called to him from the back door of their house.

"Be there is a minute," was Penn's standard reply to almost everything.

Entering the kitchen Penn headed to the sink to wash-up and along the way asked, "What are we having tonight?"

"Seafood surprise."

"Great. Wonder if I've got enough time after diner to finish that project?"

"Isn't this a place we've been to before?"

"No. Everyone I've talked to about cancer has advised the same thing, don't let cancer be your crutch for becoming in-active."

"I understand, but shouldn't you be adjusting to the realities of cancer. Like, knowing you have cancer shouldn't you be thinking of all the things you've wanted to do before its too late?"

"No. No. No.   That thinking is for people who only see a black curtain across their horizon.   I see the present and future differently."

"But have you asked your cancer how it sees the present and the future? Shouldn't you be a bit more realistic about the real state of your health?"

"Again, no. My health is fine. I have an acute challenge that happens to be called cancer. Admittedly it's a big challenge and if it isn't solved right the consequences could be very undesirable. But I am just treating my cancer as another high priority project, working as hard as possible to move myself from acute to chronic as the next step in this process."

"But are you seeing the cancer realistically? It's a life threat and a threat to our – your – family. Cancer is not just another project like painting the garage doors. It kills people and it can kill you."

"I agree with everything you just said. But suppose I went and did the things I would want to do before it's too late and did not make my cancer a high priority project? Wouldn't I increase my chances of losing out to the cancer? Or, suppose I went forward like I am now without doing those before-it's-too-late things, but engaged with others like Dr. Collins and Sari to move the needle from acute to chronic. Then, I could still do my projects while fitting cancer in as just another high priority project, goals and all."

"Right. But to do that aren't you just creating 25 hour days."

"I could see it that way if I didn't have Dr. Collins and Sari. But all that has happened up to this time has made them possible. I've learned how to be my own advocate, how to accept my life as having a permanent life threat, which we are trying to move to chronic. After all, I am willing to say 'No' to taking on one more project. And I don't want to create impossible 25 hour days.

If anything is to come out of all this it's the realization that getting the right people on the task as soon as possible – like Dr. Collins and Sari – is the best way to move the needle to chronic and defuse the stress build-up, while keeping the important things moving forward."

"So what happens if Dr. Collins decides to move-on? Then what? Aren't you back to having too much on your plate again?"

"Well, OK. Good point. I've continued to keep my list of options updated for new oncologists and treatments for my cancer. If I had to, I could switch tomorrow. Well, maybe not tomorrow. But I do know who my next go-to is and I have a list of treatment options. As the saying goes, the only certainty is change. So I am trying to be more of a manager than a worker-bee."

"OK, I can see I am not going to change your thinking. I don't agree with your approach, but you've certainly thought it through. I hope for our sake you are right."

"You're not alone and I fully understand your points. I think this is the right approach: set the goals, get the best people on the project, monitor the project's progress, and don't let it crowd-out the other things in life that are important."

"I still think you're putting too much on your plate for the sake of being busy. I think you should be making time available for us, not filling your day so you can treat the cancer as a project. You haven't cut anything out of your day either. In fact, if either Dr. Collins or Sari told you to back-off on your pace would you do it?"

"Well ..."

"Wait. What if you didn't have cancer? What if there were no life threat like cancer? Would you continue at this pace?"

"Honestly, I don't know. I do know that in the present cancer is my driving factor."

"My point exactly. I think you need to re-calibrate. You are driving yourself due to the cancer. You are not fitting the cancer into your life by getting rid of whatever you have to eliminate to make room for the cancer. You really are creating your own monster of 25 hour days due to the cancer because you would not do it if the cancer did not exist as an immediate life threat."

Standing there in silence Penn is caught in his own dilemma and has no response, but senses the error of his ways.

"Just eliminate some of the excess baggage to make room for the cancer so you also have room for us, too. You're building a stress you can't even see. That's all," as she gives him a hug and a gentle kiss.

"OK. I'll try. I really will."

WIFM - Reality Assessment #4

Some will and some won't, and I prefer the former.

Ping: *While it could be said that Ping's wife cares more for him than he does for himself, it's probably that she has seen Ping's act before and knows how to confront it. It's also interesting to observe that at times others can see through the fog of related and unrelated issues better than the cancer patient.*

While Ping is in avoidance mode, his wife sees clearly the issues Ping should be seeing and acting on for himself. She sees the consequences of his denial and that his rationalization is directly proportional to the adverse impacts of the cancer.

Net, net: Ping won more from the exchange than he will ever admit.

Pong: Obfuscation and denial are not good baggage in cancer. The PET-CT scan images are still running background in his mind as a dark cloud while he diverts his focus.

Pong's efforts to create the appearance of his being OK prevent him from seeing his cancer condition as trending toward acute, let alone ever being able to reach a state where it is chronic and more manageable.

We can see this condition mirrored in his comments about his wife's religious foundation vs. his own. While he is able to acknowledge that her religious practices have buoyed her well in his cancer treatments, he concedes that his have not. Yet, like the discussion above, he rationalizes away correcting his thinking at a time when he seriously needs to make these mental adjustments. He is not alone, we all do this. Still, two wrongs do not make a right,

Penn: Just because Penn has made a solid transition to his own chronic cancer advocacy does not mean he has his act together in all other respects. While he is engaged with an excellent team at the cancer hospital with Dr. Collins and Sari, he is in denial elsewhere.

In the previous chapter he too quickly rejected the advice of Sari to have a port installed – more on this later – while Sari knew from experience to let it drop for the moment. Professionals like Sari are able to provide insight and advice that even advocates like Penn need to heed. Either they have been-there themselves *or they have years of experience in seeing how cancer patients like Penn do themselves disservice to not accept their advice.*

Unbeknownst to Penn – like most of us cancer patients – his wife has been a silent observer of his efforts to fill his time with projects.

Her criticism is that he has become so driven by his projects - including his cancer as a project - that he has allowed no time to relax, or to be with her [they have no children].

Even in the conversation with his wife Penn worked hard to defend the indefensible, arguing against the obvious accumulation of unneeded stress. **Like the situation with Ping in this chapter, others who are close to us can often see us better than we will allow us to see ourselves.**

But, as this chapter's sub-title suggests, we all have limits that others are sometimes better able to see than we are of ourselves.

<u>*BP Score Card*</u>:
Ping = 0, Pong = 2, Penn = 0   -   In cancer friends are invaluable.
*   -   Heed the informed advice of others.*

#5 Cancer is a Disease, Both Chronic & Acute

Not going all the way? Why go at all?

Ping: Recall that Ping and his wife had made a pact that he would make a follow-up appointment with Dr. Allen if his bladder symptoms had not improved within the next two weeks. They hadn't improved, but neither did they worsen perceptibly. There was a little more of this and somewhat more of that, but the limbo status at the end of the two weeks was enough for Ping to quietly extend the due date by a month.

In his extension period, aka time of rationalized denial, Ping began to think of where he was in his cancer situation. His conclusions were less than positive, but he was unwilling to concede that his recently chosen path needed rethinking.

Concurrently Ping was not feeling very upbeat, either. His symptoms had not totally turned against him, but neither had they improved as he had hoped. They had just gradually moved him further into negative territory while he watched the movie replay in slow motion.

Then it happened, as he knew it would. His wife had never really lost sight of the missed date to call Dr. Allen for a new office visit. She finally came forward, prodding him for an update on his condition.

Ping admitted to her that the symptoms hadn't worsened much, but they hadn't improved either. If anything the intensity worsened slightly, but the frequency did not increase. When she asked how he was handling his situation, Ping said he had been taking a generic ibuprophen twice a day. And, he said, "I'm getting some relief that I didn't expect."

But the ibuprophen was just masking the problem more to Ping's disadvantage than to his benefit. A facade.

While ibuprophen is effective at reducing inflammation, in so far as an OTC anti-pain, anti-inflammatory medication is capable of doing, it is totally ineffective at slowing or halting the advance of bladder cancer. On a net-net basis, Ping's OTC self-treatment was actually worsening his condition and moving him from a relative chronic status toward an acute status because it made him feel better while the cancer advanced unabated. In short, Ping was wasting valuable time.

As Ping and his wife bantered back and forth another two weeks passed during which the pain level and the frequency increased even as Ping increased the ibuprophen to 4x per day. Finally, even he had to admit that he may be worsening his condition by further delaying the return to Dr. Allen.

At the office visit with Dr. Allen, Ping heard in more strident medical-eze from Dr. Allen how he had contributed to the worsening of his condition by papering-over the bladder symptoms with the ibuprophen because the cancer had had several weeks of re-engagement without any medical control or restraint. Together they agreed that a new CT scan would be the essential next step. Dr. Allen said he would schedule the scan and the follow-up review with Ping for ASAP.

Having been through CT scans at the same local hospital several times in the past, Ping was already on good terms with the teams and moved through the process quickly. Back at home that evening Dr. Allen called to say he had already received the radiologist's report of the CT scan and to request that Ping come into his office the next day.

The news was not terrible, but it was definitely a lot less than good. According to the report, Dr. Allen explained that Ping's bladder cancer had likely returned to Stage II. Dr. Allen continued, "We can't delay any longer. If you are still at Stage II we need to prevent the cancer from spreading to where it will have grown further into the layer of the bladder below the inner lining.

On the other hand, if it has already reached late-Stage II we need to stop it before it can spread further. In either case you must begin a new round of treatments ASAP and they will be more involved than what you experienced in the past.

Previously you received Cisplatin as a chemo therapy and it was active against the cancer. But I believe we need to go further this time and include radiation in addition to the Cisplatin. So what you experienced in the previous Cisplatin treatments is similar to what you will experience this time. But it will be more intensive. Next, because the radiation will be directed only to the bladder you will not likely have any discomfort due to the radiation and we'll monitor your progress through the entire treatment process. Are you OK proceeding with this plan?"

"It seems like I get a sequence of treatments, I get better, then it returns. Then, I get treated again. I get better again and it just never seems to end?"

"Ping, you have just described real-life with bladder cancer. More often than not, if it is not cured in the initial treatments it returns. The goal is to stay ahead of the cancer, never letting it advance to a later stage. When you delayed a return visit after you sensed a return of the symptoms you allowed it to take-off, so to speak," Dr. Allen said.

"I understand. I guess that sometimes we can be our own worst enemies. But looking back a few months, it feels like I just wanted a break at the time. Now I know the price I paid. So in answer to your question, I am OK with going ahead as you've described. Not a great choice is there?"

"These choices are never pleasant. Let's get you scheduled for your next chemo treatments and the radiation."

Pong: By now Pong had already completed the prep for his MM-013 clinical trial. The time had arrived to do what he had long anticipated. So as advised by Dr. Black, Pong arrived at the hospital to begin his new treatment protocol with the MM-013 Clinical trial. Except this time there was no Dr. Black to greet him. No Dr. Black and staff to break the trail ahead.

It was different here. In a novel way the clinical trial setting at this hospital was intriguing. The aloneness, the new techs, the staff, the new oncologists moving here and there in white coats. It was high-tech, but with the feel of being low-touch. It was devoid of the warm feeling and continuity he had previously felt on his cancer odyssey.

In the infusion chair on the fifth floor he felt like he had become a character in a Rod Serling *"Twilight Zone"* movie, but in real time with him in the starring role.

He imagined the computer keyboard's "back-key" as grayed-out and inoperable. The "esc" key was there, too, but always just out of his reach. Only the white coated staff could press it, but only at their discretion and not his. His dominant feeling was that control of his life had been transferred to others he did not know, as he simultaneously thought about words like "confidence" and "trust".

In the previous Dacarbazine treatments he had already seen the trailer to the upcoming movie, but he had not seen the beginning. First he would be hooked-up to the hydration IV with 500 ML of 0.9% saline solution. Then the preps of Zolfran, Benadryl and dexamethasone – all to quiet the nasty adverse effects of the clinical trial's MM-013 chemo.

Then the movie's pace quickened as it advanced until it was in fast-fwd and he realized this whole experience had become a game of who was killing who? But with all that toxic stuff being pumped into him by an electronic pump the size of a paperback book, it soon became impossible to tell the difference between the preps and the MM-013 chemo. It was only a matter of what bag of toxic fluid was hung on the IV pole and pumped into him by that electronic gadget?

Then it occurred to Pong, "Who were all those who had already trod these steps ahead of him. Ahh, Forget it. HIPPA rules had already eclipsed any chance of engaging them. Welcome to the next *Twilight Zone* scene."

Then there was the stream of nurses in indigo blue scrubs, all playing bit part roles. "Why can't I have a nurse like Penn's - the one named Sari?" he vexed, trapped in his IV chair.

Today Angie drew his blood to be sure he still met the standards of the MM-013 protocol. At least that was a pass. Then Susan arrived to be his nurse-de-jour. Another Pass. Tomorrow, who knows who? Then Juanita arrived to run the EKG test before they could release him. That was what she said. But what constituted a non-pass?

"In fact", he thought, "what if I don't pass the EKG? Do I become a wrong fish in the catch? Do they throw me back into the pond? Do I flounder on the roof or expire on the streets? Gee, is it actually possible to exit this place as a non-pass?"

Then, the matinee was over. It had lasted 5.3 hours. And it was over, for today. But it re-ran tomorrow. In fact, it re-ran with him in the starring role M-F each week for 3 weeks, then a week-off. A week of rest. How absurd.

Then the movie re-started. Except at each re-start he saw the same perpetually-smiling resident, but never "his" doctor.

"In fact, Pong, what are you doing? Pong, you are here to participate in a clinical trial. To kill your cancer, right? You need to stop hallucinating and get back to engaging in the trial. But am I the Pawn?" This was already inflicting perverse emotional pain on him.

After completing four cycles in the MM-013 clinical Pong was beginning, albeit slowly, to allow his sub-conscious to surface.

"Where am I? If I am the Pawn, is that MM-013 potion really killing my melanoma? After all, what's the status of my cancer?"

Then, with the force of a VW-sized asteroid hitting St. Barts point-blank, "If my smiling resident can't or won't tell me what is happening with my melanoma and if the MM-013 clinical is just a trial balloon, are we, am I, just rearranging the deck chairs on the Titanic? Am I just an understudy for Cervantes' Don Juan and I'll never …

Cervantes! Hell, this is just futility against an impossible foe? Is that why I'm cast as a bit-part player in a rhetorically supportive role to the ever smiling resident? If true, which chair was mine, and how soon? Pong, you really need to see Dr. Black again, and soon."

Leaving the hospital, Pong placed a cell phone call to Dr. Black's office. Next week at the end of his Cycle #4 was then open. He knew it was time, actually overdue, for an update. Dr. Black's AA easily scheduled Pong into an OV at 1 PM Friday.

In the OV with Dr. Black Pong began, "I am sure you have been getting the reports from the MM-013 clinical. So, how am I doing?"

"On the surface ...?"

"I see a resident who smiles a lot, but who gives me nothing. So let's dispense with the surface stuff and get to the net-net."

"OK. ... Then, based on the reports at first you seemed to respond well. In medical-eze that means the MM-013 chemo seemed to be active against your melanoma. But, then, the progress seemed to have slowed or maybe even stopped because the shrinkage we thought was occurring, well ... it appears to have stopped."

Dr. Black hesitated, recomposed himself and continued, "In fact, as a result of your most recent CT scan, which as you know is part of the MM-013 clinical protocol, the MM-013 chemo appears to no longer be active at this dosage level against your melanoma. Believe me, I am as disappointed by this news as you. I truly am."

Re-composing again, Dr. Black continued, "Today this may seem counterintuitive, but I want you to continue with the MM-013 clinical, but at a higher dosage level. Simply put, we do not have a good alternative right now and we think a higher dosage level will be tolerable and may slow or even halt the cancer's advance. I can't mandate this, but I want you to do it. I am hopeful you will agree to continue at the higher dosage level and I am committing to you that I will search every available trial and chemo for a new option."

Again, but emotionally, "Pong Can you do this?"

"Well, when the shit hits the fan and we're the only two in the same small closet I guess we both get covered together, don't we? On those terms how can I say no? If you're on-board, count me in."

"Pong, I can't promise ..."

But Pong had recovered first and cut him off with, "I can see the edge of the cliff through the fog in the distance. You've been by my side every inch of this journey and I know in my heart you are there now. Whatever the outcome I know you will be there. Let's keep moving forward, Ok?"

"Pong, I don't like this news either. Thanks for ..."

But Pong interrupted again with a wave of his hand, "You don't have to, I've learned the value of hugs."

Penn: Now in his eighth ZQT treatment cycle, Penn was becoming increasingly aware of his dependency on his team of Dr. Collins, Suzette and Sari. While he had no outward objection, he was sensing how much he had slacked-off versus his pace of advocacy before arriving at this, his latest cancer hospital. This quickly led to the singular reality that dependency could quickly evolve into complacency. And to Penn complacency was the antithesis of his chronic cancer advocacy that had so far averted his own cancer death.

He was also very much aware that realization was one thing, but doing something about it was another thing entirely.

Having fought so hard to reach this plateau, he allowed himself to admit he was savoring the inertia to prepare for the next fight and to update his options one more time.

He did not have long to wait for the next shoe to drop, but not in any way he could have possibly anticipated.

If there ever were such a thing, ZQT was a benign targeted cancer therapy. Dr. Collins had confidence in ZQT, but needed it to demonstrate it was being active against Penn's tumors, and soon.

Another PET-CT scan was a definite possibility, but Dr. Collins preferred to not put patients through a succession of scans to only see minimal incremental performance that may not be durable. The effects from multiple doses of radiation could extract high tolls on patients, too.

At the mid-point of his eighth ZQT treatment cycle Dr. Collins independently decided now was the time to act.

To date Penn could determine no shrinkage in the eleven tumors along the left side of his neck and throat. But he was equally confidant they had not grown, either. Did this mean progress, or just another false negative before the sirens went off, again? "Damn, he thought [while gripping his lower lip with his upper teeth], "I like it here and I really don't want to move again. I really want this to work."

Then, in character, but out of protocol, Dr. Collins called an out-of-sequence office visit with both Penn and Sari to explain the plan ahead.

Dr. Collins began, "I've been studying your performance in the ZQT treatment program since you became a patient here. Or, [with a smile] shall I say, since you became a patient at my presentation, then arrived for treatment. No one else before has ever done what you did to get here. Everyone else who is a patient of mine, even those who are patients here of other doctors, always follow the same referral route. But, then, you are alive and I think you are showing signs of real progress. That's what I want to talk about with both of you today and why I called you here for this office visit out of our regular sequence.

There are more things about your NHL cancer that we do not know than are known today. A lot more. But in my opinion it would be a mistake to focus on the fact that your tumors appear to not have shrunk much as the rationale for switching to some other chemo. I believe we need to focus on what has happened and why. And I believe if we do that in a pragmatic way we will soon see indications of a gradual trend toward a maintainable remission."

Reflecting on all his past treatment experiences, Penn sat still in quiet disbelief of Dr. Collins initiative and what had just been said.

"Penn, when you arrived here you were at a Stage II level of relapse and quickly on your way to Stages III and IV. While of some concern, you had already been at late Stage III when you entered your first CHOP treatments. But your Stage II at the start of the ZQT program does not begin to describe the gravity of your situation when you first presented as a patient here. And that goes to the reason why I agreed to accept you as a patient.

In our first office visit and exam I could see, even without a PET-CT, scan that you were at much higher risk than would have been indicated by the standard level of staging that was indicated by your Stage II level. You clearly had several active tumors on the left side of your neck and throat. At least three were in very high risk areas and I feared that one or two were then only about a centimeter away from being able to invade your esophagus. Were that to happen, no matter what we did to treat you, I do not believe you would have lasted six months. Which is about now.

So I had a choice. Either turn my back and not admit you as a patient because I was already in an overload condition, treat you palliatively because I was unwilling to accept the risk of failure, or accept the challenge to save the life of a very high risk patient.

Now you know why we are here, right now. But, in facts-of-life terms, if you had not done all the things you did to get here as my patient you would most certainly not be alive today.

But clearly you are very much alive. And I believe the bigger picture is what has not happened and why. If we read those markers correctly we will see the opportunity in the ZQT, and not in the rationale to quit and run."

[Hesitating for a moment] Dr. Collins continued, "I believe we need to make a few adjustments to allow the ZQT to do what it is trying to do, but is being impaired by our adherence to its standard of care protocol. First, the ZQT treatment dosage needs to be increased from 21 mcg/kg to 27 mcg/kg. Next, the dexamethasone needs to be withdrawn and replaced by an over-the-counter anti-inflammatory, like ibuprophen. Lastly, we need to be sure this stays under our scrutiny and your cancer does not suddenly take-off. I am going to engage Sari to watch your tumors closely on a schedule of Monday, Wednesday and Friday over the next two and a half cycles. So you will have to come here each of those days for the duration of this change. OK?"

"Sure. Yes. I can do that," Penn said, while looking at Sari,

"Sari, are you OK with this change?"

"Yes. I can work Penn into my schedule. Let's just be sure I know a time each day so I can add him into my schedule. Is 8:30 AM OK?"

"Good. ZQT is not an aggressive chemo. In many ways it is very benign, so we need to work with it, understand it and how it is trying to work in Penn. The fact that your tumors have not grown is the key message. Removing the dexamethasone may allow the ZQT to be more effective, especially if the ZQT is increased from 21 to 27. It will only take a few weeks of time, but these changes could produce a demonstrable improvement. Let's get started by doing an initial exam. I'll guide Sari through the steps she will need to perform and the reporting we will need."

Carefully, Dr. Collins [from behind Penn] guided Sari's fingers [from in front of Penn] over the tumors in Penn's neck and throat, adjusting the pressure of her small finger tips and assessing the relative size and location of each tumor. All the while Penn's eyes never left Sari's eyes as he kept his thoughts to himself as, "So, I've just been advised that I would have been dead by now, but instead this prettiest of all nurses is gently checking-out a few bumps in my throat. A fair trade. I can do this," Penn confided to himself.

With a glance from Dr. Collins, Sari said confidently, "OK, I can do this," much to Penn's relief.

"Good. Then as soon as you've completed each exam enter the results in a simple Excel report with each of the tumors across the top and your dated results in the rows. At the end of each week please summarize for each tumor and email the updated report to me. OK?"

"Yes", Sari said, glancing at Penn again with confidence.

Because he was then at the mid-point of his eighth ZQT cycle, Penn stayed for his regular treatment, which Sari managed just as she had all his previous treatments.

Then on Friday he returned for the exam by Sari. And again on Monday he returned for another exam, Then, Wednesday was both a treatment day and an exam day, both managed by Sari. Then another exam on Friday, also with Sari.

If there was anything adverse about this increased frequency with Sari, Penn hadn't noticed and he was not about to raise an objection.

Each of the subsequent treatments and Sari-exams proceeded as all had in the past, except each Friday, Penn would ask Sari, "Any change since last Friday?" To which Sari's dry-witted response was always, "As you know I am not your oncologist and, therefore, not qualified to advise you. You should contact your oncologist directly. Do you need Dr. Collins contact info?" After which she produced a very slight smile.

Then, to Penn's total surprise the last Friday in the revised sequence went differently. Sari had completed the exam just as she had all the previous exams.

She then recorded the results and summarized them in the report as in the past. But when Penn asked her, "Any change from last Friday?" she said, "As you know I've advised you in the past to contact your oncologist because I'm not qualified to answer that question. However, my family is from Israel and Holland - a curious mix - and we have a tradition of giving encouragement in as few words as possible. So I believe I can revise my response to your perpetual question.

As you already know I am not qualified to answer your question [as Penn's expression waxed to perplexity] and I suggest you contact your oncologist. But if I were to advise any other action on your part it would be that you should have a glass of that Sangiovese you rave about. Of course, you should always limit your intake of alcohol and consult your oncologist first. Do you understand my response?" Sari said with an expressive soft smile.

Penn was caught totally flat-footed, again, by this lady with the soft accent and gentle smile. But he was still able to mutter through a reply, "OK. I understand the first part, because I've already heard it from you several times before. You do that part well. But, the second part, the part about the Sangiovese is the part I like and don't yet understand. Could you, I mean ..."

Sari waved her hand gently, "Not allowed. Strict rules." Another smile.

"I see. OK. Sure. Makes perfect sense," Penn said recovering from his faux pas. "So I'll just have to cross the line and give you a hug, nothing personal of course. Just appreciation," Penn said with a smirk.

"Oh, OK," she said in mild surprise as they embraced.

Penn, was then sliding into emotion with the realization of what Sari had just said when he said, "I can't believe this moment. I've come all this way and I was so close to losing everything. This is the first time in almost three years I've heard anything so simple, so grounded and so positive. I think I've earned the right to say I love my team'"

Sari knew where Penn was headed before he did himself and interjected, "You're going to need some Kleenex, maybe a box of Kleenex. Just look forward to your next visit with Dr. Collins. OK?"

"You'll be here on Wednesday, right?" he asked.

"Yes, even if you're scheduled for 3 PM I know by now that you will be here at 8:30 AM. I'll be here at 8:30, too. I'll get your vital signs and send you in to see Dr. Collins. See you on Wednesday and don't forget that Sangiovese. Sounds good. Never had any."

While most people look forward to weekends for all the obvious reasons, Penn wanted this one to be over as fast as possible. Unfortunately it took the same amount of time as all the previous weekends in his life.

So Wednesday 8:30 AM arrived and Penn was already in the reception area when Sari walked-up to the reception desk. First she called "Smith", then "Rosen", then "Chavez". She turned and spoke a few words with the receptionist, then she made one more visual pass of the area, looked directly at Penn and motioned for him to follow her into the infusion area. "Damn. She knew she was going to play it this way before I left on Friday," Penn thought as he dutifully joined the end of the short conga line headed by Sari into the infusion area.

Penn's heart was already beating at 2x, but he knew she had just played all her remaining cards. Any other surprises would have to come from Dr. Collins.

Soon Sari had delivered him to the exam room and he awaited Dr. Collins arrival. Five minutes, ten minutes. Then, Dr. Collins arrived.

"Well, I understand from Sari that you are looking for an update from me about the results of our changes in you treatment regimen."

"Yes," Penn said with measured caution because he knew the news could still go against him.

"Well, if I were to summarize all of the activities, all of Sari's comments, everything over the past two and a half cycles since the changes we made, even in the absence of a new PET-CT scan, my conclusion would be that all your tumors have shrunk by about 20%, possibly more. Most important, your most threatening tumors, those being closest to your esophagus, have probably receded and are now that much further away from your esophagus."

Penn was then doing a poor job of holding back the tears in his eyes. In the space of just two minutes he had become a man who had fought a good, but draining fight for more than three years and who, at that moment, was exhausted. He had nothing left. Only emotion. Good emotion.

"Clearly, there's a lot more to be done. A lot more. We are not home free and you should know that there is still no cure for your cancer. But you are improving and we should keep doing what is working. We can back-off the exams with Sari. Now is the right time to schedule you for the next PET-CT scan. We now need it as our new treatment benchmark and to validate our recent achievements against your first scan."

"Obviously, right now I have no words other than Thanks and Thanks. I am so grateful that you and Sari are my team. I just don't know anything else to say, except that I love my team."

"I truly understand and I'm glad you fought so hard to get here. I am optimistic for your future. You should be proud, too. Let's get you back to Sari for your regular treatment, but on the revised plan. And thanks to you, too. I am sure you know that this is what I work for," as Dr. Collins reached forward to give Penn a hug.

WIFM - Reality Assessment #5

Because in cancer to not go all the way is to concede.

Ping: Cancer is a treadmill. Step off and back on carefully, else you may not like the results. *Which Ping just learned he does not like. The passage of time was fleeting, the respite of a brief remission had lulled him into a complacency that bred denial when the symptoms announced the ending of the remission.*

But, cutting Ping some slack, this is a human trait that cancer banks-on. Ping is re-entering a new-old treatment plan. Isn't it long overdue to ask, "What else is available that may be newer and more targeted than decades-old chemo with radiation? Are there others we should be talking to? Some people simply will not raise their eyes from the road, even when the pavement has ended and the road has turned to dirt. Let's keep trying, though.

Pong: *Starting his first clinical trial at the new hospital, Pong is unprepared for the new experiences. That's because he is actually in a clinical trial "factory" where he is just one of the bar coded parts.*

He is alone and in emotional pain at this "factory" because he failed to see the cancer threat early. And his doctor never looked beyond the present at any time in the past until Pong's melanoma had already metastasized to other locations of his body.

Now Pong feels the aloneness and like a pawn being moved about by others in a game where he cannot press the control keys. When he confronts the reality of the failing MM-013 clinical trial with his oncologist, Dr. Black still has no fwd-looking options.

Pong is beginning to realize the gravity of his situation, i.e. that others are playing Russian roulette with his life and he does not like the feelings.

Penn: *Put in bottom-line terms, Penn's cancer is a very nasty-bitch. But Penn made it through boot-camp in "Cancer: Who Gave Me Cancer?" and is even able to now acknowledge to himself that he is dropping his guard to not add to his list of options, e.g. who is next if Dr. Collins is no longer available and what is next after ZQT??*

Contrast Penn to both Ping and Pong who still do not even know how to ask these fundamental questions. Painful, isn't it?

*Penn can afford to savor the inertia of the moment because he has a team in Dr. Collins and Sari at a dedicated cancer hospital who have analyzed his situation and accepted the challenge against his high-risk cancer. **Penn's team is now a key and dedicated part of his offence.***

Penn's oncologist, Dr. Collins, knows the attributes of the ZQT chemo, knows his NHL sub-type, knows and trusts Sari and is willing to color-outside-the-lines to conduct a controlled test to prove that the ZQT is trying to be active in killing his cancer, but needs some adjustment in the treatment protocol. Even Sari played a key role without fracturing the rules. Hmmm, can be done!!!

So, back to the "acute" and "inflection points" questions. Yes, Ping's was a missed opportunity. Pong's was a realization that his situation had definitely made a turn for the worst and his life is now much more at risk. Yet he made no adjustments.

But Penn's was twofold: (1) not only was he not dead, but (2) his team had actually crafted a plan to improve his ZQT performance to be able to move him from acute to chronic.

So, even in cancer, this is the time to savor the moment.

Stay tuned ...

<u>*BP Score Card*</u>*:*
Ping = 0, Pong = 0, Penn = 2 – With the right team, have the confidence and let your team help drive your cancer offense.
– Always be implementing My Cancer Advocacy™ to stay on the offense.

#6   Depression & Other Facts of Life

If I could just rearrange a few of life's pages, just a few ...

Ping: It's not a great attribute of your resume to know a hospital's oncology treatment area so well that you look like you're a 20 year veteran. But that was Ping's sense going into his third round of chemo treatments. At this hospital he knew the infusion area, knew all the infusion nurses and he knew the diagnostic radiology area, too.

Unfortunately for Ping these déjà vu surroundings were unable to roust him from the depression he found himself in as he returned for his next round of treatments.

Even though his wife had tried to boost his spirits, she had to admit to herself that her efforts were not working. Ping just seemed to feel increasingly alone, even when surrounded by friends and family. He had even expressed to her that he felt more and more invisible and wounded.

Possibly his feelings were deepened by knowing that Pong was not doing as well as he had hoped for in his clinical trial. Ping had never realized till now how much Pong's journey was brought to bear on him.

Now, returning to the hospital for more treatments, especially after he had failed himself by procrastinating when he first sensed the return of the bladder cancer's symptoms, he began to sense a new reality.

His was that of an unbalanced reality of going deeper into the cancer experience, of no longer being able to see an exit back to life as it had been pre-chemo, pre-cancer. "Is this really it? Once engaged with cancer, is there never an exit? Was it just a matter of how steep the decline?" were his Sartre-like troubled thoughts.

Arriving back at the hospital for the treatments there were all the old familiar faces. At least there would be smiles and warm embraces. At least there would be a brief respite from these dark and depressive thoughts. This existential aloneness.

For this sequence the chemo treatments were scheduled to be on alternating weeks from the radiation treatments, meaning that Ping went to the hospital every week for treatments over a period of twelve weeks. Again, an endurance test.

But this time the sense of novelty had been replaced by one of resignation trending into depression. While it had its roots elsewhere, he was incapable of hiding it from the nursing veterans at his treatment hospital.

"Hey, it's Ping. Lonesome? Couldn't stay away, could you?" was the greeting from the same friendly blonde nurse in blue scrubs who had met him when he arrived for his first chemo treatments.

"Well, it's similar, but a little different this time." Ping replied cautiously while trying to smile through the reality of his situation.

"That's OK, we already know from your doctor's orders. When you walked through that door downstairs you walked into friendly territory. We even know about your radiation treatments. You're home, Ping. We make all the bad stuff go away." she said with a hug and a smile. The only things missing were the Oreo cookies and a glass of milk! But, otherwise truly existential.

Upstairs in the infusion area Ping was soon back into the familiar chemo treatment regimen. As regrettable as this return was, it was reassuring that the process was still familiar and intact from his previous experiences. But Ping's sense of this version of the infusion process was best described as being, "Off".

"Why?" were his vexed thoughts.

Was it that he did not want to be here ever again? Was it that he felt he had been betrayed about having been told he was "cancer free" or that he was harboring doubts about the whole treatment process? "What else could it be? And what the hell do I do as cancer's slope becomes steeper?"

The reality of why he was there nagged at him again and again, regardless of whether it was during the chemo treatments or the radiation treatments. It was one thing to know the reason he was there once a week for twelve weeks was to kill the cancer in his bladder. Undesirable, but understandable. Still, if the cancer returned at some time after this round of treatments had ended would he have these discomforting feelings again?

Ping's feelings of isolation did not leave him either. Especially during the infusion process there was time to think. Maybe too much time. It was during these sessions Ping tried to think through some possibilities, like getting a new oncologist, looking into other treatment options, maybe even going back to the clinical trials issue they had briefly discussed so long ago [as in Chapter 11 of *Cancer: Who Gave Me Cancer?©*].

He had come to know Dr. Allen so well that he had become his de-facto PCP, even though he was first and foremost an oncologist and not a PCP. Then, too, he had been there with him for so long. There was just so much cognitive inertia that stood against any kind of change.

He knew he hadn't done any research into the Cisplatin chemo, but he knew Dr. Allen and he just felt a deep trust that Dr. Allen wouldn't have chosen Cisplatin as his chemo treatment if he didn't have a lot of confidence in it to cure the cancer. But if there were future problems and other treatments were needed, "... perish that thought. Wonder what Dr. Allen will find to replace the Cisplatin? Must be other options. I'll just leave that to him," Ping resolved in his mind.

So, while there clearly was something bugging him about this whole bladder cancer return and the treatments, something more powerful deep inside was trying to reach-out to him in a way he could not ignore. He had finally rationalized it to being un-resolvable. Maybe, he concluded after a lot of thought, it would sort itself out on its own like his phone system at work!

After the twelve weeks of treatments had been completed Dr. Allen's AA called Ping to advise him of the need to get a follow-up CT scan at the same hospital as where he had just completed the Cisplatin chemo and radiation treatments. She also made an appointment for Ping with Dr. Allen the following week for an update office visit.

At the appointment Dr. Allen began, "Ping, it is nothing short of amazing. Your CT scan report shows no evidence of the bladder cancer. Let's hope that this time it's gone for good," he said as he conducted a physical exam during which he noted no adverse effects from the radiation treatments.

"You may feel some discomfort in the area of the radiation treatments because the tissue in that area is now more fibrous. For a while it may feel tender and like a muscle pull during exercise. But nothing to worry about. Take an ibuprophen if it bothers you too much," Dr. Allen said with the counsel of a faithful PCP. "Let's see you again in three months, or earlier if you notice any re-current symptoms. And just don't let them go on like you did this time. OK?" he said asking for Ping's buy-in.

"You bet. I've learned my lesson. Don't want to go through these experiences again," Ping said with a hint of sub-conscious doubt as if what he had just been through was nothing more than a slap on the wrist for having been too inattentive and too much his own medical counsel. Which he had been.

Pong: If Pong had looked at his options he would have quickly noticed there were two other oncologists with melanoma practices at the same cancer hospital where he was continuing in the MM-013 clinical trial. But he foreclosed all other treatment options by looking no further.

He never looked because he had never been his own cancer advocate. Nor had he ever developed his own chronic cancer options.

For Pong, the MM-013 clinical trial had become a voyage of discovery. Down deep Pong had seen the MM-013 chemo fail at a lower dosage level and was unable to hide from himself the serious possibility that it could fail even at this maximum dosage level, too. Then what?

To Dr. Black's credit, he had successfully convinced the MM-013 clinical team to increase Pong's dosage level to the maximum dose of 31 mcg/kg allowed for this dose-limited clinical trial because he saw no other option for his patient. As the dosage was raised to the maximum level he also increased his monitoring of Pong, especially for early signs of liver and kidney problems. Because the MM-013 was at Clinical Trial Phase III as a novel treatment, but with no previous experience at the maximum dosage level, it came as a surprise to the MM-013 clinical team that there were no signs of either liver or kidney problems. And the higher MM-013 dosage level appeared to actually have stalled the advance of Pong's metastasized melanoma. Were these new waypoints in uncharted territory?

Ironically, these were conflicting experiences to both Pong and to Dr. Black. To Dr. Black it was a sense of satisfaction that is more rarity than it should be in cancer treatments to gain some traction against this intractable foe. He knew that at these levels there were few waypoints pointing to positive outcomes. At least for the present he had called this one correctly.

But for Pong the present was a different experience. He was deeply grateful to Dr. Black for all that he had accomplished by going to-the-wall for him when he had nowhere else to turn. Yet, if the maxed-out dosage of the MM-013 clinical chemo began to fail there was still no replacement. This terrified him and made him feel anxious and on the edge of depression much of the time.

In a physical way Pong already knew this fear very well. He was an expert skier and had inadvertently encountered similar situations in skiing at least a couple of times in his past.

Once, while skiing in Austria, he had ventured onto terrain he was not familiar with, in part because so many European ski trails are much less marked than in North America. While he had always been able to reason his way through with his pragmatism and expert skiing ability, there was one experience he would never never forget.

For a long time he had been skiing alone at a high altitude along a long, steep trail way above the tree line. At first the trail was very wide with no apparent boundaries to either side. But, after what seemed like a strange amount of time, during which his speed steadily increased, rock walls emerged to either side of him and soon they had become very high and very steep. Just as he began to notice the height and steepness of the rock walls on either side of the narrowing trail he became much more aware of his downhill speed. It was then he realized he was a long, long way into a couloirs.

Skidding to a stop to one side of the couloirs he began to collect his thoughts, "Jesus, here I am more than three-quarters of the way into a full-fledged couloirs and I have absolutely zero options other than to go-for-it. I could be in deep trouble. It's already past mid-afternoon. There's no one anywhere near me. And, worst of all, there is no possible way of going back. None."

Looking into the découlage of the couloirs he could see almost no advantage to either side, except that the left side was in the shade of a jagged rock wall and required a jump off a cornice of about ten meters vertical drop. He knew he could lose his skis and poles, if he didn't also break one or both skis and injure himself, too.

Not that the right side was much better. It was a steep icy chute in sun that slammed quickly into the adjacent rock wall. But if he could make a very tight carve to the left as he approached the rock face he might be able to tuck into the run-out under the cornice before hitting the left side's jagged rock wall. What a choice!

"Christ, if I go right it's incredibly steep, but if it is powder under the cornice on the left I might be OK. If I can control my downhill speed, if I can keep my edges in the tight carve to the left and if I can make a hard turn to the right just before crashing into the left side's rock wall. At least the right side has some ifs."

Pong knew that to stand in the cold shadow of the couloirs' rock walls vacillating back-and-forth made no sense. He knew, too, that of the two options there really was only one and his entire future was gripped in a mélange of his perceived skill, his resolve and his fear. He continued to assess the situation as he edged backward to the middle of the découlage and onto the edge of the steep plunge to the right rock wall about twenty meters away.

Zero to 30 MPH happens very very fast on ice. For steel edges to bite into ice at that speed takes every muscle fighting for control when your skis are trying just as hard to skid-out from under you - slamming you into the rocks - then distributing your remains over a snow field as desolate as any on Everest. That's when fear kicks-in as your ally, because there's no doubt about what comes next.

Very soon after he pushed-off he leaned hard into the left turn and felt the backs of his skis graze the right rock wall of the couloirs and the intense burning of the lactic acid in his thighs and calves. Then, just below middle of the découlage the trail was less than twenty meters wide between the rock walls. But it was even steeper below the cornice before it would begin to run-out.

Fortunately he had guessed correctly, it was powder below the cornice. But now he was traveling very fast in powder as he saw the detail of the jagged rock face fast up-coming, even through the cloud of soft powder covering his goggles.

Pressing as hard as he could on his right downhill ski, he could feel the ski sink into the powder as it fought the turn. Knowing there was no choice he leaned harder into the turn hoping to only strike the wall on his hip in a glancing blow that would kill his speed, but not ricochet him down the slope and out of control with his skis and poles lost in the deep powder.

It worked. Well, it mostly worked. His skis stayed attached and his poles were still strapped to his wrists as he slowed in the steep power about fifty meters below the impact of the glancing blow.

Standing there alone and cold he ached from the impact. A glance at his suit and he knew what had just happened. As he hit the left wall, the rocks ripped his suit open vertically from his hip to his shoulder. And there was a small pool of blood forming on his left sleeve from a gash over his cheek bone. Clearly he had hit the wall much harder and more vertical than he had planned.

Still, he was alive and below the cornice. "No small accomplishment," he allowed himself to pause and reflect in that cold solo moment.

With over five kilometers of steep terrain ahead he knew this was no time to waste in self-praise as he pushed-off to the village far below.

"So, if that was then and this is now, isn't now much like then?" he reasoned. "After all, as options go I made the best of a bad lot then and it looks like I have to do the same now. And isn't cancer a lot like getting into that couloirs? Sometimes you never see it before it's already a serious threat and there's no way to turn back, much like that couloirs and how I had to make it through the best of a really bad set of options. And I did. So why not this time, but with cancer?

But what if I had crashed at that speed on either of those turns? I could have lost everything, then and there. Just like right now with everything riding on a potion called MM-013 that appears to be holding-off the melanoma's progression. Holding it off till when? Or, what if my body eventually rejects the MM-013? Isn't this really déjà vu, like standing alone in that icy découlage before I pushed-off? Or, what if the risky option never existed at all, just the cornice with that 10 meter drop? I wouldn't be here at all. I'd still be there."

By the time Pong had finished rationalizing his limited approach to the concept of his options he still felt nagged by the what-if of the MM-013 clinical chemo or "potion", as he had begun to call it. All he knew at the moment was that the MM-013 was holding off the melanoma, even if it still posed a lot of risky, unanswered questions.

To Pong it made no sense that there appeared to be no progression, but there was no elimination of the tumors either. At the next office visit he was going to press Dr. Black for what comes after the MM-013 clinical chemo. But the question of what-happens-when was beginning to generate real anxiety. "Why doesn't Dr. Black have more answers?" was Pong's new recurrent thought.

Penn: Another fact of life is that under grueling circumstances what we need and what we count on to be true and unwavering sometimes unbelievably eviscerates before our eyes. As in, "Just say this isn't happening to me."

Penn had just left his most recent ZQT treatment. His mind was still on his progress with the ZQT against the NHL cancer. And, too, on the conversations with Dr. Collins, with Sari about the port issue again, and the 'good news – bad news' lecture he had gotten from Charlie, the hospital's nutritionist.

With Sari he had heard once more about re-considering having a port installed. "Didn't she get it, I don't want it," Penn thought to himself.

But she was a determined RN. Sari also had her patient's best interests at heart and the conviction that Penn was probably fighting other concurrent, even sub-conscious, battles over the port-thing.

She knew Penn had fought long and hard to survive his cancer to this point and probably did not want to admit – at least not yet – that his NHL sub-type cancer was incurable. She believed that for Penn to accept the port was a tacit admission he would be unable to ultimately prevail over the cancer and he would see that as a failure of the advocacy he had achieved. She had already seen the same in many others and knew exactly the opposite was true, but Penn had to come to that conclusion on his own. So, to

Sari, a little patient prodding was the best course of action. Besides, it avoided an unwelcome confrontation.

"When his veins harden a little more and the IV fails to enter his veins, he'll come around," she would muse to herself as he left the infusion area.

Then there was Charlie. Charlie's agenda would have the entire planet on rabbit food, with total cholesterol below 100 and unable to get wet in a shower.

Penn had really tried to focus on her suggestions. He had gotten his glucose down to where it just nudged over the upper limit of 100 mg/dl. He had nearly switched-off of all red meat and his fluids intake was then averaging 35 oz/day. But, as much as Sari was able to cut him some slack now and then, Charlie was an unrelenting trooper, albeit for a good cause.

During today's treatment Charlie stopped at his chair while the ZQT infusion was underway, but after he had taken the pre-meds of Benadryl and Zolfran.

Penn didn't want to be rude because she was really trying to make him stronger with her nutritional guidance, but he was falling asleep as she spoke. After he awoke he remembered saying something about a "great cheesecake" at a recent party and seeing Charlie frown and shrug her shoulders. But nothing after that. Hopefully she could see what the Benadryl was doing and would cut him some slack.

Sari had been generally upbeat, but she reminded him again to think about getting a port because she was having more difficulty inserting the IV needle into his veins. Penn remembered her soft look of scold because she knew he would push-back, but she had to keep the pressure on him all the same.

At least so far, so good with the ZQT treatments. He had not yet had the next PET-CT scan, but his persistent probing of the tumors in the lymph nodes along the left side of his neck with his fingers, and the same by Dr. Collins and Sari, all seemed to confirm anecdotally that the tumors were slowly shrinking. They all knew any progress with ZQT was likely to be slow and difficult to quantify at first, but at last there seemed to be indication of progress.

He knew, too, that he would be able to shift his center of gravity back into the safety of his comfort zone once he had returned home. At least there were still places where life threats and confrontation were off limits. Or, so he thought.

Arriving home, mid-afternoon, his wife was not yet home. Not totally unusual. But she would have been more likely to have been home at that hour than to not have been home. Still, not a big deal.

Then, by dinner time Penn began to be concerned. But just then she drove her grey BMW into the driveway.

"Hmmm," Penn thought as he watched from the large kitchen window as she got of her car, "a bit dressy. Wonder what's up?"

Once inside Penn asked casually, "What's up? Anything new happening?"

While placing a magazine and her purse on the kitchen counter next to the fridge she replied with an air of detachment, "Oh, nothing new, just went to a bistro for lunch with a couple of girls from the office, got to talking too long, had a couple of glasses of wine and lost track of the time. Why?"

"Oh, Nothing. Just curious."

"Curious how?"

"Just curious, like you're dressed-up and you weren't here when I got back from the ZQT treatment. Just seemed different. That's all."

"Why? Can't I wear something different? Do I have to be here all the time?" she said still under the influence of the merlot.

"I'm just saying you seem a bit different. That's all. Nothing more."

"Well, you're different. I mean, you go off to your cancer treatments. You see Dr. Collins, Charlie and Sari. So why can't I do some different things, too?"

"Ok, but you're definitely dressed-up different from what you usually wear to the office. You have perfume on, which you almost never wear. And I've never known you to arrive home this late. So it just seemed that a few things had changed, kind of all at once."

"Hmmm ... So now I'm being monitored? Next I may have to fill out a permission slip or punch a clock. What gives you ...?"

"Why are you so uptight and defensive? All I did was comment on a few things that were obviously different about you. Nothing more.

"Well, maybe I am different. Maybe I should be. Maybe I need to be thinking more of me."

"What's that mean?"

"It means I've been thinking that I'm not sure I know where I am in this relationship. Like, where am I? Where am I going? After all, you've got a new center of gravity in your treatments, like with Dr. Collins and Sari. But where does all that leave me? It's like I don't have an identity any more. Like I'm just a tourist passing through your life. I feel invisible."

"Whoa, wait a minute. Nothing has changed between us. Nothing."

"Then, you're not able to see it from my side. You have changed by the cancer and this relationship has changed, too. They're not the same and they're not going where I thought we were going. Like I said, I feel like I'm invisible. Like I'm just a housekeeper. And now I feel like I'm being monitored and that I may need to punch a time clock."

Shaking his head "No" Penn said, "No. No. No. Not true," but she cut him off.

"Yes, it is true and I'm beginning to feel like I need a break so I can figure out who I am because I thought I knew..."

"A break from what?" as Penn cut her off.

"I need to recalibrate."

"You need to do what?"

"I need to understand how things have changed, where am I in these changes and how am I affected? What are the impacts on me? After all you had to go through the same process when you learned you had cancer."

"I can't believe I'm hearing this from you...

"Why, because I'm always here for you so that you have come to take this relationship for granted?"

"Where are these ideas coming from?   Is there someone else who is putting these ideas in your head?"

"Wait a minute. Just stop right there. You're going down the wrong road."

"Right road, wrong road, everything was fine this morning before I went to the hospital. Then, fifteen minutes ago you walked into the house somewhat late, all dressed-up like you had been to a party, wearing perfume that you almost never wear and claiming you feel like a tourist in our marriage.   Certainly it's not unreasonable for me to ask what is going on. Don't you think?"

"Well, maybe it's just been coming for a long time."

"So, is there more?"

"I'm sure there is more, but I don't know what at this time. I do know you've changed, like from the treatments. I know your focus is now the hospital, Dr. Collins and Sari.   And I do not feel as though I have a role anymore."

"Huh? Changed how?"

"Like look at all your treatments. You've been through so many of them. What have they done to you? What happens to me?"

"You mean sexually?"

"Sure, that too. Like how does it affect me? I need a timeout to think this relationship through. I really think I do."

"Gee … I never saw this one coming. But, you sound like you have something in mind. Do you?"

"Uh, but first you need to know and understand there is no one else. If that's what's wandering around in your head, forget it. Get rid of the idea because it's not true. I am just thinking that I need a break for a while because I just don't know who I am anymore."

"You don't know who you are anymore? Am I missing something here?"

"Like, I want to go for a visit to my sister's in Charleston."

"Ouch."

"You're doing fine and you're making progress. You've got Dr. Collins and Sari. Besides, all our conversations begin and end with them anyway. They might as well be here now. I'll just be a cell call away. I really want to try this. You need to give me a break."

"Honestly, I never saw this coming. I'm truly sorry."

"I know you are ... can you?

"Sounds like you're firm in this. Obviously, I think I need to..."

"Thanks," as she reached across to give him a hug, but no kiss.

WIFM - Reality Assessment #6

If only it were so simple...

Ping: *Is this the best there is available?*

Clearly, Dr. Allen has done little to benefit his patient past the most rudimentary treatment plan. It is devoid of any knowledge as would be available from a PET-CT scan and it fails to consider more contemporary chemos. One can readily see how the stage is being set for another round of treatments when his bladder cancer relapses, yet again.

And what about Ping's lingering state of depression? After all, it is possible that his depression is attributable to having no options in either other oncologists or chemos. That is, without options he is painting himself into a corner of diminishing returns. His inertia is preventing him from doing what he should do, i.e. see cancer as a potentially chronic condition and become his own cancer advocate.

In other words, even at this date, after having completed three treatment plans, Ping still does not know what he should know. And that can hurt him. Like, are there other less toxic treatments for his bladder cancer? Are there other oncologists who are more experienced with less toxic treatments? What newer clinical trial options are available? Again, he doesn't know.

These options are critical because options are patient-facing and forward-looking. Cancer doesn't sleep and it adapts. He's dropping the ball on his own "My Chronic Cancer Advocacy" at a time when he could be moving forward into a durable chronic condition. **In cancer options are the antidote to depression.**

Pong: Pong's situation is a lot more tenuous than Ping's. His melanoma has metastasized, he is already at the maximum dosage level for the MM-013 clinical and he is treating the MM-013 chemo as a life-dependent drug, not as the marginal clinical chemo that it is.

Furthermore, Pong has just rationalized his cancer treatments against a previous life threatening challenge – much as any of us could against comparable challenges – and missed the essence of that challenge relative to his cancer situation. He needs to STOP. Get a grip before it's too late. But it's not happening.

First, the MM-013 chemo is only believed by Dr. Black to be "...holding-off further progression of the melanoma". Is it, really, and how validated?

After all, the MM-013 is not yet a commercially available drug, nor do we know what is meant by "...holding-off further progression of the melanoma", nor has Dr. Black come forward with one or more alternatives to the MM-013 drug.

So, while Pong is motoring along, his melanoma tumors could be growing in-situ, or preparing to spawn newer tumors. And, as yet, he has nothing to replace MM-013 if it fails to "...hold-off further progression of the melanoma".

Pong's comparison of his cancer situation to the skiing experience missed the point that there were two skiing options, but especially in melanoma he needs more. He missed that he, Pong, failed to notice how he had created his own life threat by being inattentive to the changing conditions. And he missed that his skiing skills were what enabled him to cheat death on a ski slope. But melanoma does not play by the same rules, i.e. his skiing skills are useless against cancer because he needs the skills of others to prevail against his cancer.

Pong is missing that MM-013 bought him time, like Penn's clinical trial experience in Cancer: Who Gave Me Cancer?©. He has to be his own advocate to locate a successor to Dr. Black and the replacement(s) of MM-013. Pong is at an inflection point.

He needs more treatment options and he needs a new oncologist who specializes in melanoma. And he needs both very soon because the melanoma will not suffer these errors without extracting a very high price.

Penn: *Heads-down, totally focused on his cancer, his projects and his team of Dr. Collins and Sari – as he needed to be as his own*

"My Chronic Cancer Advocate" - Penn never saw what was happening around him until it was too late.

His wife had supported him and, while he hadn't rejected her, he hadn't valued her. And that can be both risky and painful, especially when you are on the receiving end.

It is probably even more difficult for Type-A people because they have a greater propensity to charge ahead, blinders fixed in-place and unable to have any peripheral vision in so far as others are concerned until the crash occurs. This can be especially true for those of us who have such life threats as aggressive cancers that we are able to exclude everything that is not on our daily critical path.

Penn had already encountered this issue when his wife challenged him previously about his 25 hour days, but he blew that off then and so missed the coming storm.

His wife said she was going to her sister's in Charleston, but Penn never got a full accounting of the perfume issue.

Let's hope Penn hasn't begun to conquer one problem in his cancer, only to lose a valuable resource in his wife.

<u>BP Score Card</u>:
Ping = 0, Pong = 0, Penn = 0 – *Mitigate the depression of cancer by always being on the offense.*
– *Part of having a cancer offensive strategy means always having options.*

#7 Hello, Big Picture

All the world's a stage.

Ping: Ping had struggled with his return to Dr. Allen, struggled with his return to a third round of treatments for his bladder cancer and was doing his best to keep the whole matter to himself while he continued to see each incident as an event unto itself. Kind of like dots are just dots.

The problem with all his heads-down focus was that he saw each situation in isolation, not as part of the big picture of him and his cancer. In fact, for Ping there was no big picture.

Each dot, aka experience, was just that, a dimensionless dot with little or no impact from the previous and none to the next. Was it fear, obstinacy, denial or maybe procrastination? Whatever "it" was, "it" was not halting the forward advance of his cancer, because cancer doesn't sleep or cut deals.

Sure, in the office where Ping worked most of the workers knew of his cancer problem.   But they mostly afforded him the courtesy of privacy. Yet, every now and then someone would ask, "How are you doing?" to which Ping would routinely fend-off the question with an "OK" or "I haven't had a problem in months" to avoid other more probing questions.

In truth, the reality was different because beneath it all Ping rejected connecting cancer's events into a picture of any kind, let alone a "Big Picture". To Ping events were events. Sure, events could eventually become a bigger problem, but that was later, much later. Maybe never. And to Ping dwelling on events was better left to others. Like the details of his health insurance, as in chapter 10 of *Cancer: Who Gave Me Cancer?*

One day at the office a woman from HR asked him, "You're looking great. Are you now over the cancer and don't have it any more?", as though they had not seen each other in the three years since he had had his last treatments.

Ping's response was just as emotionally neutral, "I haven't had a problem since about a year ago, so I may be cured."

But, of course, the most recent bladder cancer treatments had just ended a few weeks earlier, not "about a year ago". While the incident might otherwise be lost to passing conversation, it's important because Ping intended it to be just that, lost to passing conversation.

Where it could have been a benchmark of, "Did anything happen today that I need to make note of for the next appointment with Dr. Allen?" it became lost to unrecorded history.

Ping did not maintain a cancer journal for the same reason. That is, journals record events and events lead to more events which lead to problems. So no journal, no events, no problems. Believe that at your own peril!

While this logic worked for Ping, much like his PCP - ala OCP - logic in Cancer Who Gave Me Cancer?, it was nothing short of frustration for those who cared most about him, like his wife.

That evening, after the non-event conversation with the HR woman at work, Ping and his wife were discussing the upcoming Christmas holiday over diner of her homemade spaghetti and chianti, as in what gifts to get for who and what parties to attend and which events to decline. Ping's wife was a quiet, pragmatic Italian woman who picked her important moments carefully.

"So is this our list of friends and relatives? Any others we need to include?" Ping said with a glass of wine in his right hand while holding the list off the table with his left hand.

"I think that's it. I wrote it this afternoon, trying to pull it together for tonight. Is there anyone I might have missed? I didn't include the kids because we always do them together anyway."

"This works. Can we get started this weekend?"

"Sure. But are you OK? I mean have you had any new symptoms?" she asked in her soft probative voice.

"I'm OK. Why do you ask?" Ping asked with a slight hesitation,

"I just want to be sure going into the holidays."

"Nothing new to report."

"Nothing?" she said with a little more edge to her voice and a casual glance that said she knew more than she was willing to share at that moment.

"Nothing. Well, maybe a little more frequency. But why?" Ping said defensively, as though he had been caught with a cookie in his pocket.

"Because I've noticed."

"But it's nothing. Really nothing to make a big deal over."

"But frequency has always been a marker for the bladder cancer's return. Why not now?"

"Because it's just a little more frequent, and not even that much more frequent."

"But isn't frequency part of the bigger picture that first its more frequency, then it's a small pain, then its …"

"No. No. It's just a little more frequent and not even that much more frequent. Maybe just a little. That's all. Why do you have to fuss over it more than me?"

"Because I don't think you see how these events or symptoms can be part of the larger picture."

"Look. A little more frequency could be for a lot of reasons other than cancer, like for foods or fluids. So how does that cause me to have more cancer?"

"Maybe it doesn't, but if you stopped the foods or the fluids the frequency should stop and I haven't noticed that, so I'm thinking that maybe …"

"You're thinking I have more bladder cancer because I just have a little more frequency. Nothing more. No bigger picture. If it pleases you I'll just plan to go less frequent."

"You know that's not what I mean," she said in frustration.

"Maybe. Maybe not."

"Whatever you're thinking just stop thinking those thoughts. It's just that I've noticed your more frequent trips to the bathroom and I'm concerned. Just like the last time and I'm concerned that the problem could be creeping-up on you again."

"OK, I hear you. But I'm OK. Really. There's no pain, no other symptoms, no bigger picture. Can you just drop it? Just stop putting me under the microscope. OK?"

"Probably not."

"No?"

"Right. I think there are two problems here. First, you don't see small events as symptoms that can lead to bigger symptoms, then to bigger problems. Second, you don't see your bladder cancer in a big picture way where small events eventually become bigger events that become bladder cancer. You only see bladder cancer as bladder cancer when it has become a big life threat. At other times you're in denial, at least till the freight train runs over you at full speed."

"Not true."

"Is true. Happens so often you can't see it any other way. You're just hurting yourself and us."

"But a little increase in frequency is definitely not bladder cancer."

"Really? Then how does bladder cancer start?"

"Look, I don't have more bladder cancer. I just want to stop this conversation about my cancer and get back to where we started about our Christmas shopping. Can we just do that?"

"OK, but I still think you're making a big mistake to not see small symptoms like increased frequency as a possible part of the larger picture, because you could be seeing the symptoms return very early and head-off more difficult treatments in the long run," she said with the determination of an attorney making a closing argument.

"Got it. Moving on. Can we get back to the Christmas list thing?"

Continuing with the conversation Ping jumped in, "Oh yes, listen to this, today at work the HR lady in the office told me about how taking asparagus was supposed to cure cancer. I thought I should give it a try. Hey, might work," Ping said to close off her "Big Picture" discussion and switch to a less challenging topic.

"Whatever. But do you now want to have asparagus on your eggs in the morning, as in eggs-ala-asparagus?"

"She said I should have it three times a day with regular meals."

"Right. Pureed, poached and fried?"

"Didn't get that far. Does it matter?"

"What matters most is that you begin to see your cancer in a bigger picture."

"Will you stop with the bigger picture stuff? Maybe I should try the asparagus ..."

"You'll never change," she said in exasperation as she headed off to the kitchen with her glass of Chianti.

Pong: As a heads-down engineer Pong saw the world in terms of dots, as in files with of lots of dots needing analysis before the files could be forwarded on to others who performed more work on the dots. So, too, he viewed his cancer as a file of dots. And he could see how the dots could be organized into files, even collections of files. Yet he failed to see – for his own heads-downness, lack of vision, in-attention, you name it – that in cancer the dots and clusters of dots were themes and members of a larger story then playing out inside him. After all, his job-job was all about the analysis of dots.

To Pong the events of his cancer were dots, too. But, just as he seldom looked past the interpretation of the sequences of the data dots in his work, he saw the events - dots - of his cancer experience, analyzed them to discuss as dots and passed them onto Dr. Black for him to take to the next level of assessment and disposition.

More important, Pong never differentiated the dots of his work place activity from the accumulating events of his cancer. So he failed to see the worsening message the cancer was sending him over time. The "Big Picture" was, and had always been, the agenda of others.

While this placed a big burden on others, especially Dr. Black, it also meant that Pong was unlikely to ever see his cancer goal in the context of a chronic condition, let alone the acute condition that was advancing inside him. And it greatly compromised his ability to become his own advocate. Too bad he never connected these.

Even others could see this in Pong, much like we can see ourselves in the mirror, yet not see what we do not want to see. Dave from work was a friend who liked Pong and just had a hunch there was more to Pong's cancer story than maybe even Pong was himself seeing. Dave had been thinking of approaching Pong about his friend's health status.

On a calm Wednesday afternoon in December with no threat of rain Dave just knew in his soul that he needed a solo bike ride after work, but before dark could settle in. So he left work a little early to get to his bike at home. Heading out he made a couple of quick calculations, deciding to only do a quick 15K loop up thru the oaks and pines to end-up back at *"Un Bel Di"*, his favorite café-bookstore overlooking the park.

"I could do this ride a thousand times and still see something new and beautiful every time, just incredible. Should have invited Pong, but he has something else on his mind and probably would have declined anyway. Hope it's not more to do with his cancer," Dave was thinking as he reached the crest of the ridge, about 10K into the 15K ride.

The rest of the ride was down the slope's run-out and across the toe of the slope, then through a fragrant eucalyptus grove and back into town by about 4 PM. That still left plenty of time for a pre-dinner snack at *"Un Bel Di"*.

Un Bel Di was a former commuter railroad station of old brick with a slate roof at a small park surrounded by tall pines where the tracks had once been. It had enough room to house a small bookstore. The café just added ambience to *Un Bel Di's* charm. Then, having the best coffee and pastries just ensured a steady competition for reading space in its few isles and at the small a-duet marble-topped bistro tables in the café and on the outside terrace.

Pretty moms with an open agenda usually made it by mid-morning. Then, the local professionals arrived for lunch. The afternoon was always a mixed-bag of moms toting pre-school kids, out of work CEOs, and neo-literates looking for the next great read. Other types not fitting this description were always welcome, so by mid-afternoon *Un Bel Di's* cafe was an eclectic collage of patrons with interrupted agendas.

Knowing it would be cooling down on his return, Dave had scrunched a fleece pull-over and jogging pants into the bike's sack to be put on at the end of the ride. So walking into *Un Bel Di* he just looked like every other late afternoon patron.

Picking up his cappuccino he turned to survey the available tables in the café when he noticed Pong looking back in his direction. "Hey dude, seeking new literary insights? What brings you here?" Dave asked while strolling over to Pong's table. "Is it OK ...?" Dave asked from a few feet away.

"Yes. Of course. Please join me. So is this what you do with your sick days?" Pong said with a smile as he cleared away an area for Dave to place his cappuccino.

"Well ... look who's talking, I mean it is only 4 and the office still has another hour ..."

"Uh ... right. I just needed a break. Like you?" Pong backhanded to Dave with another smile.

"OK, you won that serve. What's up?"

"Nothing really, just an hour before getting back into regulation home life."

Dave offered a look of questioning disbelief, then, "More health problems?"

"No big events. Nothing like that. Just thinking about events, how they happen, what causes them, what I could be doing. But, truthfully, there's nothing going on."

"You mean like 'How Did I get here?' Or is it something else?" Dave asked with a bit more probing voice.

"Nothing dire," Pong said, holding his real concerns to himself.

"Are you thinking you need to go beyond your current plan? Maybe a second opinion or more treatment options?"

"No, no. But these things puzzle me. Dr. Black is doing a fine job.

He calls all the shots and has made so much progress. Don't want to think of questioning him. I just don't understand these few events that don't fit with the rest of the progress."

"Do you think you need to step back to take another look, like at the big picture?" Dave said carefully, sensing that he may be pushing the edge of Pong's protected limits.

"Good question, but that's Dr. Black's space. I don't go there. He knows what's available as far as all the treatments. I don't. He knows this far better than I ever could. I couldn't start second guessing him now. Couldn't do that. Wouldn't go there," Pong said with a hint of defense.

Knowing he had reached an impasse with Pong, Dave took the last sip of his cappuccino and checked the view out the window, "Hey Dude, it's getting really dark and I still have a 2k ride to home. Got to be moving on. See you at work tomorrow, or should we meet here?"

"Great idea, but I'll be at work after my doctor's appointment. Thanks for listening. Glad you stopped by," Pong said still with his head pondering his original question about how and why his dots, aka events, respond the way they do.

"I'm glad I did too," Dave said as he got up from the table with his empty cup, but a little disappointed he was not able to alter his friend's head-down focus, even just a little. Dave knew Pong was not seeing the big picture, but was at a loss for how to get his friend to lift his eyes from the minutiae to the bigger picture.

Next morning, before going to work Pong headed to Dr. Black's office for his scheduled appointment. At the OV Pong asked all the same questions as he asked in the last OV, and the OV before that.

And Dr. Black responded with the same answers from the previous OV's. Meaning, he had not identified any more promising treatments to replace the MM-013 hold-over from the clinical trial. And he was not seeing the melanoma spread. But without a new CT scan he said he could only comment on what he saw in today's physical exam, and that he did not know why Pong was experiencing different rates of healing at the sores on his back. He especially could not explain why Pong was getting sudden sharp pains that quickly dissipated.

"Let's not wait any longer. Let's get you into a new CT scan to see if there is new activity since the last scan, something that might shed some light on your issues. It's a little early and there's no major event taking place, but I can argue your need for this scan with your insurance carrier if I have to. If we can schedule you for the scan this week are you available in the early AM?"

"I'll make the time available. Go ahead. Just leave a voice mail on my cell phone for the date and time. Thanks," Pong said, relieved of the feeling that the ball was no longer in his court.

Penn: With his wife now out of their house and at her sister's in Charleston, Penn's new cancer life was more different than he could have imagined. That is, had he imagined it at all when he fait-accompli agreed to the separation.

"Damn, this is not what I wanted. Not at all. No one to talk to. No one to be close with. The cancer. The pains. I mean, like no one at all," Penn thought to himself in that empty space that is filled with aloneness and physical and emotional pain.

"If I call her I'll sound weak. If I ask her to come home I'll sound like I'm giving in. And she could easily say 'No'. Then, I'd be worse off than I am now. Yet, if I continue talking to myself like this soon I'll start answering back. Then, I'll be in even more trouble. What a pit."

Still working on his solo conversation Penn reasoned, "The large tumors in my lymph nodes still hurt. Actually, they hurt a lot. There's a treatment tomorrow. Then I have to go till next Wednesday before the next treatment. That means the pains in my neck and throat will be worse than now by the weekend and there will be no one here. Damn. Solo in cancer sure is hell."

"Can't call Sari or Dr. Collins. That's over the line. Don't want to call friends for a beer because the pains will still be present and I'm no good at hiding that stuff. Don't want to burden them either. I've been here before in this disease. I can tough-it-up. I'm going to have a glass of wine, watch a movie and go to bed.

I'll be there for the ZQT before 8:30 AM. Early, but not too early."

Indeed, next morning at 8:30 Penn was in the hospital's reception area waiting for Sari. But the pains in his neck – left side and under his left jaw – had greatly increased to where he was barely holding back the tears. Sari's arrival at the reception desk was as welcome as it was possible to be.

Quickly, Penn completed the vital signs routine and Sari had him seated in his favorite infusion chair. She had promised to get him started on the pre-meds, but the infusion area had quickly become very busy and Sari had no spare time to spend with him. The pre-meds did not happen as planned.

As she attended to several other patients in the infusion area the stinging of the greatly increasing pains in his neck and under his jaw could no longer be ignored. They were going beyond intolerable with no hint of peaking or backing down.

After a few more minutes in silence he could not hold back any longer and the first few tears slowly fell from his eyes, across his cheeks and onto his crossed arms, leaving large dark wet spots on the front of his blue shirt. Then more tears and more quickly. Then more, but at a pace that raced ahead with the increasing pains. Slightly heads-down, unable to stop the onslaught of the pains and unable to halt the tears, Penn suddenly felt totally alone on that foggy, dark cliff again.

"Where does this stop? Has the ZQT finally lost the battle? Is this the end, again?" as his mind raced into those darkest of corners.

"Hey! Hey, Penn! Look at me. It's me, Sari. Take these tissues. I'm sorry to have left you here in this much pain. I'm really sorry. Please forgive me. Please?"

"Damn, she even had tears in her eyes," Penn thought as he peered at his pretty nurse through a flood of tears and his aloneness began to ebb.

"I'll be back in two minutes. Just keep mopping," and with a brief clutch of his left shoulder she was gone.

But she really was back in two minutes. Sari was back with two pills with, "Here take these with this cup of water."

"What are they?" Penn asked, interlaced between a pair of snuffles.

"Never mind. Don't ask. Besides, Suzette will just have another fit. The day's already headed in that direction anyway."

"Is the ZQT finally starting to fail?" Penn asked with a solid hint of resignation.

"Of all my patients you should know more than anyone that it can't fail if you don't have any in you. And here I thought I had been working with better cerebral material. What are they going to send me next, another tourist?"

"But ...," Penn tried to interrupt.

"Look at your cancer and the tumors this way: If someone was holding your head under water, wouldn't you kick and scream to break free? Of course you would and that's what's happening right now in your tumors. The ZQT has been doing a great job of attacking your tumors. But you have several very advanced tumors. There is a major battle taking place in you right now. The tumors are fighting back, but they have no chance against your ZQT treatments because they have no defense against the ZQT as a targeted therapy. What feels to you like you are losing the battle is actually you winning the battle, but the tumors will fight back the only way they can. Right now you're caught in the middle. The big picture is that you're still acute, but our goal is to get you to that land of chronic maintenance.

Right now that may seem like a moon shot to you, but the ZQT is going to win by killing the tumors. You'll see." she said with the confidence of a young mom who had just put the idiot-mittens back on her young child for the fifth time that day. Sari knew the big picture with absolute clarity. And she knew there could be no big picture without details like the idiot-mittens routine.

Penn continued to look at her in quiet disbelief when Sari asked, "Are you beginning to feel less pain?"

"A lot less. What was in those pills?" he asked.

"Best to think of them as a secret potion for special patients. Just keep your eyes on the big picture, just like you did to become a patient here. Don't lose that heading and we'll take care of the details. OK?"

"OK, but it's been a long time since I've had an attack like that."

"I understand. I've hung your pre-meds and the ZQT will be here soon. Just lay back and rest. Think big picture and I'll take care of the sun-block. OK?"

"Will do," Penn said as he lay back and closed his eyes with the pre-meds beginning to course into his veins. Within a few seconds he was soundly asleep.

Then, right on queue Sari was back gently rubbing his arm to wake him. "You're all done. We don't have overnight accommodations at this hotel."

Rousing himself from a sound sleep Penn asked again, "What was in those pills?"

"Forget the pills. Just keep your compass set on that horizon and I'll see you again next week. You sure you're OK to drive home?"

"I'm Ok. I'm going to get a mocha. Thanks."

"You and that mocha thing, again. OK. Bye," she said as she placed her steadying hand to the small of his back as they walked past the nurses' station to the reception area.

But instead of heading to the garage and his car, Penn veered off to the cafeteria for something bearing a large amount of caffeine and a snack to replace the lunch he had slept through ... courtesy of Sari.

Amazingly, the severe pains of only five hours ago were gone. With a mocha and a scone in hand Penn was headed back toward the infusion area, then to the garage, when he saw Mimi coming in the opposite direction from only about ten yards away.

But she looked different. Something about Mimi was very different. Penn could see her mom was holding her arm so as to steady her.

Penn needed those ten yards to gather his composure because Mimi did not look like his Mimi. She was thin, gaunt, even ashen, with her beautiful eyes now more deep-set than ever.

There being no more distance Penn wanted to reach out to embrace the person who had meant so much to him in those early chemo days, but Mimi gently stepped slightly aside.

"Mimi, I can't believe you're here and with your mom," Penn said, trying to hide his shock and knowing the news was not going to be good.

"Penn you look great. I've been through an allogeneic stem cell transplant and I'm struggling with some immune system rejection. I'm so tired. Believe me I could use a hug right now, but I can't get too close. Let's just set a rain date. OK?"

"I understand. I'll ask Sari to put us on the calendar. Will Sangiovese be OK?"

"Penn, you know I'm Italian. Sangiovese will be just fine. Be well and don't forget our date," she said very tired while her mom gently led her away.

But, until he re-connected with Sari, Penn knew there was no way he was heading toward the garage. None. Zero!

Instead he headed back to the infusion area in search of Sari. But just before he could re-enter the area Sari intercepted him.

"What the hell is ...?" Penn said, emotionally very rattled.

"I just caught a glimpse of you two. When I saw Mimi here earlier I just knew you two would happen. I know how much she means to you, so I wasn't going to tell you for a while ... till we could see how she handles the anti-rejection meds. But when I saw her here today my gut told me a collision was going to happen. I'm so sorry."

"But, that wasn't ... I mean it was ... Damnit Sari, what happened?"

"Mimi has had an allogeneic stem cell transplant. She is just now able to be out of isolation, but very carefully. She now has someone else's immune system and her body is not doing as well as we had hoped at accepting her donor's immune cells," Sari explained patiently to Penn.

After a moment with Sari holding Penn's shoulders she said, "We have her on anti-rejection medications, but she still does not yet have a fully functioning immune system. Not yet. And she's really struggling right now."

"Can we just go back and replay this movie and leave out all the bad stem cell stuff?" Penn said, still very upset.

"I know how deeply you hurt for her right now, but for Mimi there was no choice. Unlike you, Mimi had reached that point ... she had no other options. Believe me, there were none. You're part of her big picture right now. Just do her a big favor. Send her a nice card, but no flowers because she can't risk an infection. Do it from both of us, but don't put my name on the card. Just sign it 'Penn and a Friend'. OK?" Sari said looking intently into Penn's watery eyes.

"Yes, sure. Will you get in trouble for telling me about her?"

"Maybe. About the same as for those pills. I know how much she means to you and how this has really shattered you today. We're all a lot more fragile than we are willing to admit. Again, keep both big pictures in perspective and try to be there for her as she has been there for you. Now it's Mimi who needs you."

"Damm, I was so totally heads-down into my own stuff. I never saw ...," Penn said in painful reflection.

"Unfortunately it's too routine at places like this. Count yourself very lucky. Are you OK now?" Sari asked.

"The card is on its way," Penn said quietly.

"You got a mocha, didn't you?" Sari asked with a smile.

"You noticed?" Penn said with a little more life to his eyes.

"Whatever else I do, I know when someone like you gets it," Sari said with an embrace.

"How can I say thanks?" Penn said.

"Just get that card for Mimi before you finish your mocha. OK?"

With a silent "Yes" nod, Penn headed off to the hospital's boutique and away from the garage.

WIFM - Reality Assessment #7

Keep the big picture in perspective.
Sari

Ping: *Some people never get past the dots in life, regardless of the context. For some, like Ping, dots will always just be dots. Even for those who lack a life focus, it's still not OK.*

This can be a risky, self-defeating proposition because the two are in direct conflict with each other. Coasting through life may be an acceptable go-fwd plan to some like Ping - not mine - but, it will not work with cancer. **Cancer patients need to have a plan with attainable goals because cancer never sleeps. Never.**

Pong: Like Ping, Pong is disengaged from the decision making in his cancer treatment plan, even though he relies on his work methods as a de-facto guide in his cancer management program. This reinforces that one size does not fit all.

Because he has failed to become his own chronic cancer advocate he has also failed to develop a plan, i.e. a sense of the big picture with the dots organized to achieve the big picture objective. So when challenges occur he has no frame of reference. This toxic combination can be very undesirable and difficult to reverse.

Even while our supporters see our missteps, like Dave, as cancer patients we need to be open to their perceptions. **Without a big picture plan and the dots organized as tactics, the best efforts of our supporters are likely to go unheeded.** To our detriment.

Penn: In cancer, life can come at us very hard and Penn has just been hit hard twice on the same day.

Sometimes as rugged as we think we are, we learn that we are all actually quite fragile.

The pains in his neck were the instigators of the rapid onset of doubt that caused Penn to lose focus and begin questioning his treatment regimen. The combination of the pains and the doubt led Penn to question his strategy, i.e. his own big picture. When that happens to us it can be quite easy to second-guess the legitimacy of our big picture and tactics.

The big picture is the strategy, the goal. Absent such a destination, in cancer we can too easily wander away from our plan. That's when our team is so valuable. In times of stress and doubt they can keep us focused on the big picture and headed in our own "My Chronic Cancer Advocacy" direction.

Recall from "Cancer: Who Gave Me Cancer?" that as a nurse Mimi had had a lot of medical training, but Mimi had never actually developed a sense of her own "My Chronic Cancer Advocacy".

Also, that Mimi's cancer is actually curable. But even a curable cancer can get away from us. That is how Mimi ended-up, as Sari said, "Unlike you, Mimi had reached that point where she had no other options. Believe me, there were none."

It's a very important reminder that when our backs are against the wall in cancer that we've likely already exhausted our best options.

Being on the offense with a goal like "My Chronic Cancer" and tactics of "My Cancer Advocacy" are the best ways to avoid having only a bad lot of options when the worst happens.

One of our most important achievements in cancer is to have troops like Sari on our team, reminding and supporting us to stay the course. They help us keep that big picture goal of chronic cancer advocacy always in our focus.

BP Score Card:
Ping = 0, Pong = 1, Penn = 1 – "My Cancer Advocacy" is a collection of dots we assemble into "My Chronic Cancer", like an impressionist painting is created from dots of paint into a beautiful picture. Same is true for our BP Score Card.

#8 Heroes

Not everything that is faced can be changed,
but nothing can be changed until it is faced.

Ping: Having gotten up early for the long drive to a business meeting, Ping now had the same long drive home to think over the day's meeting. Like what had and had not been accomplished?

Soon his mind was wandering, but not out of tiredness. The meeting had been another of those that every meeting-ologist advocates against. It covered the firm's current products – like no one knew the current products; it covered some new products – the ones everyone already knew were not new; and, lastly, it covered recent changes to the employee handbook – as if everyone in the room was not already asleep by now anyway.

If there was a positive side to the meeting it was in getting the regional team together in one place for a cross-functional event and a working lunch over pizza and soda. Everyone was in violent agreement that the pizza was great – again; the garden salad could have come from any salad factory – but absolutely not from any legitimate deli; but, the brownies and cannoli were totally landmark and legalized the meeting. Besides, it's a recognized medical fact that calories, cholesterol and carbs make great bonding agents that no comatose meeting agenda can dislodge.

So, interspersed with the camaraderie of another gourmet lunch with his long-time friends and co-workers, Ping's thoughts wandered back to his cancer situation and what he thought he knew vs. what he did not know about his cancer.

Ping knew there were a lot of things he did not know about his cancer and even more that he did not want to know – including that he did not want the cancer. Period.

Still, when you're alone on a long drive over open Interstate roads and you have cancer there's not much more to think about. So you do.

At the very least it was still clear to him that all the other people he had encountered with cancer – especially those who had lots of medical specialists – they did not appear to be any better off than him with just Dr. Allen as his oncologist. Even as they argued the case for their army of specialists, Ping rationalized to himself while driving that they were no better-off in their cancer than he was in his. "Makes no sense. So why change?" he muttered into the dashboard of his SUV with a faint right-handed wave from the steering wheel.

"Then there were those educated cancer elitists who not only had lots of specialists, they had their heroes too. Where is this going to end?" he concluded with another so-so wave as he continued into the late afternoon's reddening sunlight.

"Heroes! And how are heroes going to alter my cancer? Just something more to get in the way. Nuts. Just nuts.

Nuts ... yes nuts, as in food nuts. That's right, I almost forgot that I'm batching-it tonight. It'll be dinner time soon and I'm solo tonight. I should treat myself to dinner-out. Like "Café Soleil" would be a great treat and maybe I'll run into someone I know. Good idea Ping. Just do it. OK. Done," were his comments to himself as he began to veer away from his thoughts of the cancer stuff.

Walking up the steps to *Café Soleil* there was a cool breeze from the north making its way through the park. The evening breeze gently swayed the branches of the tall pines making it too chilly to linger in the park or on the terrace of the café. Inside it was warm.

Café Soleil's warmth was beguiling because its presentation was upbeat casual, not pretentious. Its walls were of light colored elm veneer woods and large mirrors. There were not too many tables so as to make for difficult conversations. The kind of spot where Ping quickly felt comfortable over one of his adult beverages.

Just after ordering a gin and tonic Ping noticed a familiar face a few tables away. The man and his wife, most likely his wife Ping thought, were just finishing their coffees and had just paid their bill. As they arose from their table Ping's glance made eye contact with the man, with the pleasant surprise of a familiar face from his past.

Ping recalled him as his English studies professor at that two year college he attended after high school. Simultaneously searching for his name, while remembering the English studies classes, Ping quickly recalled his name as that of Professor Albert Aaronson.

Professor Aaronson stood out to Ping from his many other instructors, including those from his aborted studies toward a four year degree, because he seemed to have so much more teaching ability and charisma than the other instructors at that two year school. Even as a two year college instructor in English studies Professor Aaronson already had a PhD. He had published papers on Conrad, Sartre and Kafka – so, why was he still teaching at a backwater two year college? Ping failed to see the rationale.

Ping learned that he had come to America as a young child of parents who had emigrated from the Safad area of Israel. They had seen the tensions building in an area that had long been a crossroads of Arabs, Israelis and Christians. They thought their young family would be happier and more secure in America.

In his classes Professor Aaronson was engaging, even with those students who more often seemed could not care-less about the course's content. They just wanted a passing grade at the end of the semester. He never picked a fight, but he often tried to engage his students to get them to think about how others had handled life's challenges and how they had prevailed over very difficult situations. A tough challenge.

Professor Aaronson knew he wouldn't be able to get all his students to read books like Conrad's "Lord Jim" or Faulkner's "The Bear" or to engage on artists like Escher or Cézanne. But he still tried to get them to see the problems others had faced as life's experiences so they could see how they had been there before them and had prevailed.

He seemed to add a special spark and intellect to his classes without being arrogant.

Maybe he already knew he had a special gift to reach those who he intuitively knew were not likely to go beyond a two year college education. To give them something they could rely on down the road. Unfortunately not all his students got the message.

Ping found his classes engaging, but only to a point. He just could not see the need to delve too deeply into what seemed like a story's hidden meaning. Like, who cared about a road not taken in a Robert Frost poem? Was it really worth spending an entire class on such a simple decision? Or what was the big deal about a boy trying to find a bear in a Faulkner story? After all, how were these pieces of literature going to be useful beyond being just another read?

As Professor Aaronson and his wife approached, Ping stood-up and offered a handshake to his old acquaintance.

"Wow, how long has it been?" Ping said with a welcoming smile.

"Yes. And under very different circumstances. You're looking well. What are you doing these days?" were the opening lines from Professor Aaronson.

"I'm doing well with just that two year degree you helped me earn. I am married and we have a small family. Been in the same job for a few years. I'm batching it tonight because my wife is out with the girls," Ping said with a hint of pride.

"And, this is my wife Beth," Professor Aaronson said.

"Pleasure to meet you Beth. Are you having dinner and would you like to join me?" Ping offered.

"No. No. Just finished. We're off to do some grocery shopping, then stop to see a friend who is under the weather. Just thought we'd catch a quick dinner first. Enjoy your dinner. Nice to see you. Hope our paths cross again," Professor Aaronson said as he and Ping shook hands again and they turned toward the door.

Pong: It's interesting how two friends can see the same subject so differently, yet seem to see it similarly to outside observers.

In Professor Aaronson's classes Ping had the opportunity to see how others had prevailed over their adversities, but he rationalized them away in favor of his own myopic perspective. On the other hand, Pong saw the possible value of heroes through a distorted lens that prevented him from reaping real value just when he needed it most. Still, to outsiders acquainted with both they came across as the same result: rejection. In reality these different means of rejection could have the same devastating effects.

In relative terms Pong's cancer situation had actually worsened because the MM-013 clinical chemo had declined in its effectiveness against his advancing melanoma. But, just when Pong should be aggressively advocating for his own cause, i.e. his life, he was frozen in inaction with no frame of reference so that the present moment became a template for all his future moments. Whereas Penn went into his P3 Clinical with his eyes wide open: if it didn't kill the cancer, then he would use it to buy him the time of transition to the next chemo on his list.

Like the moon is tidally locked to earth and always faces the same way, Pong's dysfunctional ideology is preventing him from acting on the failures occurring in his treatment plan. In fact, as time ebbs away and the news becomes more adverse he avers on key decision points of his team, his treatments and overall progress against the relentless melanoma. To recall Churchill: "We placate the alligators in the false hope they will eat us last."

Late one afternoon, while on a casual walk through the town park, Pong's path crossed with that of Rev. Buehler from the church Pong attended infrequently. Rev. Buehler had left the church, which was on the hill above the park, and was more on a mission than was Pong. He was headed to a meeting with other local clergy that included a rabbi, a Catholic priest and a Muslim Iman. They all met frequently to discuss contemporary issues confronting their religions.

"Well, it's Pong. It's been a while since I've seen you in church. I am hopeful all is well with you?"

"Yes, all is well. But you may know I've had a health challenge for a while. I seem to be holding my own," Pong said with a hint of defensiveness because he had not been to church lately and he knew Rev. Buehler likely knew of his health issues.

"I heard from a couple of others in the congregation of your health problem. Come. Sit for a few minutes [as Rev. Buehler sat down on a park bench]. Please tell me about the problem. I truly care about all of my flock," Rev. Buehler said in a soothing tone and a hand to Pong's shoulder.

"It's been a long journey," Pong began, "I have melanoma. Maybe got it as a kid and it's taken this long to reach its present state. I've had some surgical removals of the melanoma from my back and I've had a few chemo treatments, but the latest clinical trial may be reaching a stalemate. We just don't know where it stands at the present time," Pong said with the relief of having someone to talk to in confidence about something he had so steadfastly kept bottled-up within himself for so long.

"Pong, I sincerely want you to know that you are in my prayers. Do you have a good oncologist?" Rev. Buehler asked.

"I do," Pong said, not wanting to reveal Dr. Black's identity. "I have been in a clinical trial for the past few months and my oncologist is looking at the next options to succeed the current clinical trial in the event we need to find a replacement."

"It certainly sounds like you're in good hands, but keep in mind that others have faced difficult challenges such as yours and were able to prevail over their adversities because they had role models," Rev. Buehler said.

Pong sensed this conversation could be headed into well charted waters of heroic characters from the scriptures so he said, "Yes, I keep a close watch for those as guide posts while I stay close to my oncologist for the next treatment option," knowing that the former was a prevarication of the truth.

Looking at his watch Rev. Buehler said, "Pong it's been great to catch up with you and I pray that you'll soon emerge from this health challenge stronger and wiser for the experience. I have a commitment in a few minutes at the local synagogue where a group of us from three other religions talk about contemporary issues.

I'm going to use our conversation to discuss the role of heroes as role models in life's challenges. Our encounter has been very fortuitous. Be well and please try to come to church," Rev. Buehler said as he rose from the park bench and they parted with a hand shake.

Watching Rev. Buehler walk across the park Pong thought to himself, "Sure, but what hero saved Jesus after he was betrayed by Judas?" as he confused the role of intervener with hero.

"Besides, heroes are for people with more time than I have. I need a solution and only Dr. Black is going to have that answer on what to replace MM-013 with next. Now is clearly not the time to change horses at mid-stream," Pong concluded as he left the park bench and continued his walk to Dr. Black's office.

In the office visit Pong told Dr. Black that he was feeling generally OK, but he had had a cold – with mild congestion and a cough - for what seemed like a long time and with no response to a few over-the-counter cold medications.

Dr. Black advised Pong that at this moment he had no immediate successor to the MM-013 treatments Pong was continuing to receive, but said, "I am pursuing two possibles and should have an answer very soon."

Next, he said he wanted to be sure the cold meant nothing more than just a simple infection and he would send a prescription to Pong's pharmacy, but before taking the first dose Pong should do an updated CT scan, preferably tomorrow.

Because Dr. Black had been so pro-active about the new meds and the possible replacement of the MM-013 clinical trial chemo Pong was actually eager to go for the next CT scan. After all, this was even better news than he could have hoped for after the rather depressing conversation with Rev. Buehler.

Then, late that same afternoon Pong received a call at home from Dr. Black's office. The CT scan had been scheduled for the next day at 10 AM and to not eat anything after 10 PM that evening.

As had been his experience on all the previous CT scans, he filled out the same questionnaire as he had before, drank the contrast fluid as he had before, had the IV contrast line inserted just as before, laid on the CT scanner table and slid through the scanner's donut hole. Same as in all the previous scans. Nothing unusual, even the same chit-chat with the techs running the CT scanner. So there seemed to be nothing to be concerned about.

About 4 PM the day after the CT scan Dr. Black's AA called and left a voice mail message while Pong was out. He was to call Dr. Black's office for an appointment as soon as possible.

"Gee, did the CT scan get messed-up or maybe even lost? Then, again, the CT scanner could have broken during the scan and they didn't find out about the failure until the radiologist attempted to read the scan for a report to Dr. Black. Damn, just hope I don't have to redo the scan," he thought.

Next day Pong went to work, but told his team he had a doctor's appointment and would have to leave early for a 4 PM appointment across town. To this non-news event no one seemed to even notice because people just always have personal things they need to attend to, sometimes spontaneously.

Later in the day as Pong sat in Dr. Black's examination room his mind was on an intractable engineering problem at work. Seemed that no matter how much heads-down focus his team applied to the problem, it just remained an unsolvable show-stopper. Then, one of the team members suggested an internet search to see if other engineering teams had solved a similar problem. The rest of the team applauded the idea and that is where Pong left his team as he headed out to the appointment with Dr. Black.

Pong was eager to get the appointment with Dr. Black over so he could get back to his team before they left for the day to see if their new - outside the lines - approach had yielded any new solutions to the engineering problem. While he waited in Dr. Black's office it became clear that the doctor was busy with other patients and the time was fast approaching 5 PM, time for the engineering team to head home for the day.

So Pong made a cell phone call to his team leader for an update. While his team leader had already left for the day, his lead design engineer said they had not gotten the problem solved. But the internet search had yielded several responses from other engineers and the team was going to stay a while longer to investigate the novel ideas. He sounded excited and made the call shorter than Pong had expected.

Next, Dr. Black's nurse arrived and showed Pong into an empty exam room. Alone, Pong thought to himself, "More waiting. I'm anxious to get back to work."

Just then Dr. Black walked in, but not with his usual friendly smile. This time his face was more sober looking. Not terrible, but not his happy face either.

Dr. Black quickly began, "Pong your latest CT scan is back and I also have the radiologist's report. His review of the scan indicates two small masses on your lungs, one on the right lung and one on the left lung. Both being accessible for surgery or radiation. I see that you're a non-smoker, but did you ever smoke? [Pong shook his head - No] The radiologist's thinking is that these masses may be new tumors from the melanoma and that it has metastasized.

His report goes on to say that after he located the two masses he went back to the start of the review to see if there might be more than those two. He confirmed that he could locate only those two small masses, but advised that he was unable to determine if there had been any activity in any adjacent lymph nodes. I have your CT scan on my computer and you can see here [as Dr. Black pointed to the computer screen with Pong's CT scan displayed] to where the radiologist located the two masses on your lungs.

By the way, metastasized melanoma often shows up this way, as tumor masses on the organs. But more often they are not discovered until much later, so we have reason to believe we found them very early. Your cold may have helped you more than you might think right now.

Next, I called the radiologist to discuss the report directly with him. I wanted to know if he had any doubts that there could be more masses. He said he was reasonably confident that the masses were metastasized melanoma. He said he was unable to find any other indication of the melanoma having spread further at this time, but had some concern for possible spread to your lymph nodes.

Pong, clearly this is not good news but it is not as bad as it could be either. That would probably be the case if we were to find it later. It's also too early to say that your cold is related to the masses on your lungs. Much more important is the determination of what to do next.

I've had a conversation with another oncologist about your cancer and this CT scan and we've agreed on a treatment plan. Are you OK with what I've said so far?" Dr. Black said in anticipation of Pong's response.

"I understand. I sure don't like the news, but it's not totally surprising either," Pong said with a noticeable hint of displeasure. He knew he had reached the destination that was the result of not having a replacement for the MM-013 clinical chemo earlier.

"OK. Then lets continue," Dr. Black said to keep his part of the office visit moving forward.

"Having already been through surgery, two treatment sequences of Dacarbazine as standard chemo treatments and the MM-013 clinical we are leaning away from more Dacarbazine chemo because it's not getting the job done. Instead our thinking is for a combination of Interleukin-2 and radiation treatments. The Interleukin will be administered much like your previous chemo treatments. It's intended to stimulate your immune system to attack the cancer masses on the lungs and any that may be in your lymph nodes and to increase the effectiveness of the radiation treatments that will follow the IL-2 treatments.

Unlike surgery, radiation has several benefits and few, if any, adverse effects. With the chemo treatments, once you've had a chemo sequence it's possible to develop an intolerance to the chemo. That may have happened with the Dacarbazine.

That's why we want to use IL-2 this time. But radiation can be re-applied and we will get to see quickly if the cancer is responsive. So if you're agreeable we can proceed quickly, which is what I recommend," Dr. Black said in conclusion.

Pausing for a moment to assemble his thoughts Pong said, "So you're advising a sequence of the Interleukin treatments and the radiation treatments. Right?"

"Correct," Dr. Black confirmed.

"OK, then I have a question. Will we be scraping the MM-013 clinical?

"Yes, we will be stopping the MM-013 clinical because the melanoma has metastasized and the MM-013 is no longer being effective in your metastasized condition. We want to increase the effectiveness of the radiation treatments and to do that we need to attack the cancer with a chemo-like treatment that stimulates your immune system. Because you only appear to have two small and accessible masses on your lungs we will be able to see the treatment results quickly. The side effects of the radiation will be almost un-noticeable to you.

Then, in the event we need additional treatments, we can repeat the radiation whereas repeating the chemo treatments is more problematic," Dr. Black said to move the discussion away from more conversation about alternative chemos because [really] he had none at that time.

"OK. I see. Then, let's get going on the combined treatment plan.

Who do I have to see and what do I have to do next?" Pong asked.

"Good. We think this is the right next step for you. I'll make plans for you to begin the Interleukin treatments and arrangements for you to meet Dr. Bernstein who will develop a radiation treatment plan. His office will be in contact with you to set up an appointment.

Dr. Bernstein is located in this complex and is well respected here in radiation treatment of melanomas like yours. While you'll be seeing him for the radiation treatments, I'll continue to see you as your oncologist and for the Interleukin treatments so there will be no interruption in your care," Dr. Black said to wrap-up the office visit with Pong.

Penn: Meanwhile, unlike either Ping or Pong, Penn had had a much more pro-active engagement with his cancer. He had settled into an active routine with the ZQT treatment regimen and the team headed by Dr. Collins and Sari at this, his fifth hospital. The routine, if it could be called that, had begun to take on a personality all on its own with his new temporarily-permanent life style.

With his wife now into a part-time job near her sister's in Charleston, Penn's life had changed, like a rug being pulled from under him as he watched in silent protest. Although their marital separation was only supposed to have been for her to get a break, it had taken on a kind of permanence they had acquiesced to and for which there was little further discussion between them. It just happened.

They just seemed to accept it as the evolving decline of their marriage, both of them trapped by Penn's inability to be cured of the NHL cancer and his wife unable to reconcile her place in the marriage. So the separation took on a life of its own as it motored on without either a map with waypoints or a destination.

Just as nature abhors a vacuum, so do estranged relationships.

Into his personal vacuum Penn sub-consciously inserted his ZQT treatment regimen as he began to treat the entire ZQT treatment experience at the cancer hospital like a new second home. Instead of looking forward to coming home to an empty house, absent of conversation and activity, he turned inward in his search to learn more about his NHL cancer and his thoughts ranged beyond the next ZQT treatment.

This created a horizon to look forward to and a definition of the intervening time into which he could plan out his other tasks. "Isn't it queer how cancer has its own way of redefining a busy person's time while creating its own priorities?" Penn would often think to himself.

With the next ZQT treatment set for tomorrow Penn had already begun to prepare his to-do list, who he would be seeing, what he would say about his most recent NHL symptoms and any adverse effects from the last ZQT treatment, what to take for reading materials, what to ask Sari and Dr. Collins about the tumors and when they might be gone and so forth. He also thought a lot about Mimi and if there was a slim chance of another encounter. But, after her stem cell transplant, another encounter with her was so unlikely that he did his best to not dwell on the thought too much, lest it become a disappointment when it didn't happen.

So, just before going to bed, he set out all he would take with him next day. Even his routine had become a routine unto itself.

Arriving at the hospital next morning a little earlier than usual with his well-worn leather carry-bag slung over his left shoulder, Penn could have easily passed for any other medical student. He just looked the part. Except that his cancer made this cancer hospital his new second home in a way that no university with the ultimate transition goal of graduation ever could. As much as it had become his de-facto second home, his team had become his extended family.

Soon he had cleared the reception desk and there was Sari waiting for him, much like a pre-school teacher looking after her little people, like they were her own because they needed so much special care. Which they did!

"What's new?" would be Sari's opening line. And it was.

But, just as in the past treatments, she was on to the next part of the conversation before Penn could say, "Same old ..." So, Penn said, "Same old ..." but paused for Sari's inevitable interruption.

"Dr. Collins won't be here today due to an off-site conference. Suzette will cover for Dr. Collins and sign the orders for your ZQT treatment, assuming your blood work is OK. Haven't been up to anything strange, have you?" Sari said without ever looking into Penn's eyes as they walked to his IV chair from the vitals area.

"I'm solo these days, so life's been a bore. Only an occasional glass of wine," Penn replied.

"Since when is a glass of wine boring? Never mind. I'll pass your nouveau condition on to Suzette. She's already married and maybe she'll have some ideas that I wouldn't," Sari said in one of her dry quips of humor.

"I've drawn your blood and you're all set with the hydration. Suzette will see the blood results in about a half hour and in about an hour I'll be back with your pre-meds. Suzette will stop by before she approves your ZQT order, but she is incredibly busy today with Dr. Collins away. Charlie is here today, too, and will probably be by soon. Let her know about your new wine addiction, but avoid the solo stuff. I'll check back in a while," Sari said in that soft accent, while pushing the service cart into the adjacent supplies staging area.

"Hey. My hero. You're looking great. Long time, no see," was not atypical of Charlie when she was in an upbeat mood.

"Not sure about the hero thing, but this team has made a huge difference. After all, I'm alive and able to have a glass of wine now and then," Penn said swatting the verbal volley back into Charlie's court.

"Actually, yes to being a hero. People like you have somehow figured out how to get here against all the hurdles. You're right about the team here. But if you hadn't figured out how to prevail over your cancer through so many show-stopping obstacles your team would not have mattered. Please allow yourself some hard earned credit. Wine is OK and medicinally approved, too," Charlie said with the determination of a litigation attorney making a key point to the jury.

"OK, you're right. I guess I've earned a glass of wine," Penn said after being pushed to the ropes by Charlie.

"I've looked at your blood work and your vital stats over the past several weeks and you're doing well. Your cholesterol has come down nicely, but you are still too heavily into the ice cream. I can tell because your triglycerides are higher than we'd like to see them," was Charlie's challenge.

"Well, I ...," Penn started to say.

"Sari told me you would try to deflect me away from the triglyceride concern by telling me about having wine to balance the ice cream. Won't work with me. I'm not about to lose one of my heroes to a stupid blood clot. But, seriously, try to put more balance into your meals to lower your triglycerides. OK?" Charlie said with her hand to Penn's shoulder and one of her "I care about my patients" smiles as she moved on to her next patient.

After another ten minutes Sari and Suzette arrived together, Sari with his pre-meds and Suzette to quickly review his blood work. "Your blood work looks fine and I've signed your ZQT order. I'm very busy today so I'll leave everything else to Sari, but have Sari page me if you need me for something urgent. You're looking very much improved over your arrival here. Seems like this is becoming a way of life for you, isn't it?" was Suzette's stoic parting comment under Sari's watchful eyes.

Almost an hour went by and Sari was back with the ZQT and a second nurse to be sure that Penn was Penn, standard precaution in the administration of oncology treatments. But by then the Benadryl had begun to make Penn very drowsy. Soon after Sari started the ZQT IV Penn was sound asleep. Still, unbeknownst to him Sari kept a constant watch over him as she attended to her other patients.

By the time his ZQT infusion was ending Penn was beginning to awaken and Sari had just arrived to silence the pump alarm lest it wake him. Just then all three arrived at the same place at the same time.

"So I hear you're one of Charlie's heroes. Got any yourself?" Sari inquired while tending the IV pump.

"Sure. Why do you ask?" Penn said.

"Oh, just curious because you seem to take the entire process different from others. Maybe it's personal. You don't have to answer," Sari said with a hint of defense.

"Not a problem. Really, it's not a problem. Just that no one has ever asked, that's all," Penn said.

"Didn't mean to …," Sari started to say defensively, but Penn waved his right hand to cut her off.

"Really, it's OK. I'm not sure how others look at this, but mine are big people. People who were challenged by big issues or events and stood up to their situations at high risks to themselves," Penn said.

"Like who?" Sari asked.

"OK, there are eight: John Kennedy, Winston Churchill, Golda Meir, Lincoln, Colin Powell, Stephen Hawking, Gandhi and a lady named Helen Nearing. You probably never heard of her," Penn said on an up note.

"Uh, OK. But why them? And Helen Nearing. Never heard of her," Sari said while pre-occupied with Penn's IV lines.

"To me they're people who accomplished great things against incredible obstacles. I call it bravery of the heart. I greatly look up to all of them and hope to aspire to even a small piece of what they achieved, but I've got a long way to go. Helen Nearing is a long and personal story," Penn said while watching her complete the infusion process and detach the IV line.

"Well, here you go [as she placed a bandage on Penn's arm where the IV needle had been]. Please send Mimi a cheer-up card from both of us. Just sign it 'Penn and a Friend'. Don't forget, you're her hero. OK? See you next week. Dr. Collins will be here then, too," she said while pushing the service cart away.

On leaving the hospital Penn felt strangely odd, even somewhat aimless with Sari's last words still ringing in his head. With his most recent ZQT treatment behind him, no wife at home, no interest in returning to his job at mid-afternoon he just felt, well, aimless. For a while he thought about a sail on his small sloop, *Sueño*, but in the end he decided on a short drive along the coast to find that card for Mimi.

As enjoyable as the drive was, it was both a little too familiar and over too soon. His singular accomplishment was stopping at the general store in a small coastal farming village on the chance of finding a nice cheer-up card for Mimi. Mission accomplished. Penn knew he still needed more space, so he decided to take the winding road up from the coast and back into town. "Maybe a few moments at *Un Bel Di* will be enough to interrupt this malaise," he thought.

Even for those with nothing to do there's always something in slow motion to watch at *Un Bel Di*. So with no Sari or Charlie present to scold him, he ordered a café mocha and a chocolate biscotti.

Penn opted for a table on the terrace overlooking the comings and goings at the center of town. By late-afternoon the encroaching fog made the terrace a solo patch of sunlight to watch school kids, a few moms with strollers and a few job seekers checking out help wanted ads on their tablets over their day's last coffee. But overall there was no one he knew. "Probably just as well," Penn thought to himself.

Using the moment to sign the card to Mimi, "Penn and a Friend", while otherwise aimlessly pondering his café mocha and the chocolate biscotti that he dipped into the mocha, he was unaware that Dr. Collins had just entered the café from behind him.

"Hi Penn. I saw you sitting here just staring off into space and I thought I should say 'Hello' and offer you my apology for not being at the hospital today for your treatment,' Dr. Collins said.

"I understand. Not a problem. Please join me," Penn said while gesturing to the open chair at his table for two.

"OK, but for just a moment. I have another commitment, so I can't stay long. I understand from Sari and Suzette that your blood work was fine and the ZQT treatment went well," Dr. Collins said making small talk.

"Everything went well. But after finishing the treatment I couldn't figure out what I wanted to do with the rest of the day, so I just wandered and here I am. Still with no answers. I guess I'm trying to figure out what happens next if I am able to at least reach some kind of Mexican standoff with my cancer. I had been running so hard for so long that I think I'm finally starting to catch-up with myself. Make any sense?" Penn asked.

"First, I like the chocolate biscotti, but what is that you're drinking?" Dr. Collins asked before answering Penn's question.

"Café mocha. Keeps me awake after the Benadryl and pre-meds. Sari gives me a hard time about it. But I just think she's jealous," Penn replied with a smile.

"She probably is jealous, but your secret is safe with me.

Back to your question. It makes a lot of sense and I often see it in others, but not always with positive results. Sometimes people lack the ability to see how their lives have changed and they just become stuck in a perpetual malaise, unable to see their other opportunities beyond the cancer experience. Unfortunately it happens too often," Dr. Collins said.

"Not that I'm there yet, or that I will ever get there, but do you see that happen even in those who have been able to reach some level of chronic treatment maintenance?" Penn asked.

"More often than you would think possible. While cancer is a very threatening disease, it can also be a chronic condition. I wish more people would see it that way. And a lot of people lack points of reference by which to set their goals, so the cancer becomes their own personal black hole. It sucks in all their energies and creativity. I've even seen situations where that experience has accomplished what the cancer was unable to achieve. It can be very sad,"

"Then where do we break free of the malaise and into a new life?"

"Good question. From my experience those cancer patients who are most successful are not necessarily those with the biggest egos, or with the most religious zeal or even the most money. They're those whose course is set on a distant horizon and, surprisingly, those who have long standing heroes, as waypoints, who have overcome big obstacles in their own lives,"

"You mean ..." Penn started to say.

"Right, and much like you had a goal to reach a cancer hospital like ours and no one was going to stop you. No one and nothing. Remember? But when you reached that goal you did not re-set to a more distant goal and I think that's where you are finding yourself now. My guess is that you're a person who does have heroes and you are mentally beginning to re-connect with the support of your heroes who've faced daunting obstacles and prevailed,"

"So, you think ....," Penn slowly verbalized his thoughts.

"Yes. I see you doing that now. This is off the record, but I understand you've had some personal setbacks and I certainly understand your current cancer situation, so I think you're going through that cognitive adjustment process now. If you don't mind me asking, who might be your heroes – assuming I am right that you do have heroes," Dr. Collins inquired.

"Yes, I do. Well, since you asked they are Kennedy, Churchill, Lincoln, Gandhi, Golda Meir, Colin Powell, Stephen Hawking, and a lady named Helen Nearing. Why?" Penn asked.

"I don't know of Helen Nearing, but as a peer of the others on your list she must be someone I should know more about. That's an incredible list. Just incredible,"

"Thanks. I didn't see it that way," Penn replied.

"Don't treat yourself so hard. You're doing much better than you think you are doing. My suggestion is that you follow your café mocha with a glass of wine. You should be proud of what you've accomplished. You're on the winning team.

Here's an idea for you. Think about what comes next in your life, not about the next ZQT treatment. Think beyond yourself and what you've learned in your struggle against cancer. You might find that you are able to grow by helping others in similar predicaments, and your heroes will no doubt continue to support you."

"Maybe you're right. Life's been difficult lately," Penn reflected.

"Oops, I'm going to be late. Have to get going. Seriously, think about that glass of wine. See you next week,"

For a while longer Penn just sat there solo in his late afternoon, absorbing Dr. Collins candor at his now half empty two-place table on the terrace with the fog relentlessly encroaching closer. Finally, the fog's chill overcame the café mocha and it was time to move on.

Leaving the terrace he headed back through *Un Bel Di* on his way back to his car when he encountered Sean from work just emerging from "*Aqua Caliente*", the local Mexican watering hole also known as "*Hot Waters*".

"Hey, Penn. Great to see you. Weren't at work today were you? Missed you. I'm about to head home to the missus, but I could be talked into another pint?" Sean said in an obviously happy state.

"Love to Sean, but I'm headed home too," Penn said, mindful of the old axiom to never let an Irishman buy your first pint, especially if your first pint would obviously be his fifth or sixth.

"Got it, Penn. They've got the Irish football game on the tube here at *Aqua*. [Sean hiccups] Man, all those guys are my heroes. I know all the Irish teams [Sean hiccups again]. Got any heroes Penn? [third hiccup]" Sean says with a little more volume in his voice.

"Sure, like Churchill," Penn said.

"Ahh ... can't do Churchill, Penn. He was a Brit. Can't do Brits as heroes Penn. Can't do that," Sean declared to Penn.

"I can see your point. I'll give it some thought. Hey, I'm going to be late if I don't get going. See you at work," Penn said while reversing course to beat a hasty retreat away from Sean and the possibility of more encounters like Sean at *Aqua Caliente*.

On a more direct route back to his car Penn reflected on the conversation with Dr. Collins, that maybe he is in better condition than he has been willing to give himself credit for.

Passing a mail drop, Penn sent the cheer-up card on its way to Mimi, while briefly reflecting [with a soft smile] on Mimi and how Sari had inserted herself into their lives one more time.

On the drive home Penn thought, "Maybe a glass of wine is the right thing to do, even if solo at home. After all, at home there will be no chance of another encounter with Sean or any of his buddies.

Besides, soon I'll need to counteract the café mocha if I am to have any chance of sleep tonight!"

WIFM - Reality Assessment #8

Still, even cancer is not invincible to change.

Ping: *Just gotta wonder about some people. If a terrorist had a gun to your head would you be thinking of your options or making small talk? Ping has such a gun to his head [or more appropriately to his bladder]. But as much as he dislikes having cancer he's not making progress, just making small talk.*

Ping rationalizes away the progress of others who have both cancer specialists and their heroes as the domain of those "educated cancer elitists". If others have preceded us and successfully prevailed over their obstacles, wouldn't it be a worthwhile endeavor to benefit by their experience? Especially against such a determined adversary as cancer.

Encountering Professor Aaronson, Ping failed to see Prof. Aaronson as a role model for overcoming obstacles, or to learn from the success of others. Even if the person is not your hero at least let their success contribute to your progress against the cancer. In this way Ping is paying a big price for the loss of something that is free.

Pong: *Like Ping, Pong rejected the concept of heroes, but not out of Ping's myopia. He rejected them because he perceived it wrong to switch horses at mid-stream. He mistakenly confused heroes with interveners. These are important errors because they can have big impacts on outcomes.*

Even when his engineering team got the collaborative help to solve a difficult engineering challenge [albeit by a non-affiliated engineering contact over the internet], Pong was curious about the outcome, but not the means his team used to address the problem.

This should have been a wakeup call, but Pong is still asleep at the switch. He is unable to see that others have prevailed over these problems before him. ***Our cancer problems need not be faced alone.***

Because cancer never sleeps, Pong is starting to pay a price for his accumulating errors. The metastasized melanoma is the price of compounded errors. Versus either Ping or Penn, this is a turning point in the road. In the long run, with cancer "luck" is a fickle and capricious ally. Durable heroes as combat hardened veterans are more worthy allies.

Penn: Although Penn's cancer situation is slowly improving, he has not had a free ride. His newest solo status is not without strings attached. He is still very much in the clutches of his NHL blood cancer and his hard fought past is now playing catch-up with him.

But, compared to either Ping or Pong, he is more open, more organized and more resilient. Like when Dr. Collins engaged him in conversation at "Un Bel Di", he actually listened and we can sense the gears meshing in his thought process as Dr. Collins explained the value proposition of his heroes, reinforcing even his own conversation with Sari earlier in the day.

Against the odds, but in synch with his strategic goal of "My Chronic Cancer" and his tactical means of "My Cancer Advocacy", Penn is making forward progress as he learns to always be on the offense.

Sometimes, too, we overlook how our seemingly small achievements, i.e. as in gradually prevailing over our cancer problems, can become a goal setting experience for others. We often fail to see them because we're too close and too engaged as it happens.

Notice, too, that unlike either Mimi or Charlie, no one has anointed either Ping or Pong as their hero. Both Prof. Aaronson and Rev. Buehler are still advocating that Ping and Pong buy into the concept of heroes while Penn is much more advanced.

As for the encounter with Sean, well fortunately Sean's heroes are not Penn's heroes.

BP Score Card:
Ping = 0, Pong = 0, Penn = 1 – Heroes add humility, perspective and lift when the road ahead looks to be dauntingly impossible.
And, their free.

#9 My Cancer Never Sleeps

In cancer you can do or do not, but there is no try.

Ping: Like many of us, work for Ping was a reflection of how he ran his life. His work was a means to earn a wage, to support his life style, to provide for his family and to build a comfortable future. While this description could be applied to most of us, for Ping and others like Ping in cancer it also held a deeper meaning.

Ping did not see his job as fungible, but it was. His job was secure so long as his employer did not view outsourcing of jobs like Ping's favorably. Yet, Ping contributed to his marginality by failing to increase his own value. In effect Ping had taken the easy road and had failed to add value in his job as the world changed around him. He was marginalizing himself and he was becoming replaceable.

Even when the conversation turned to cancer there was a reason why Ping's glass was often half empty. Over time he never developed the means to fill it and this impacted his sense of worth.

Ping was a follower, not a leader. More often than not Ping took the path of less resistance. As in the selection of his health insurance policy, when he allowed a clerk with less competency in health insurance than himself to be his guide on such an important decision.

So it should come as no surprise that Ping acted at the direction of others and only provided back to those others the information needed to maintain his status quo and little more. No insight, no analysis, no forward thinking. As such, Ping was like many workers who allow themselves to become expendable commodities by failing to invest in themselves so that they become their own dead ends.

While he was friendly and well liked, Ping failed to advocate for himself – just treaded water - so he never advanced to where he was part of a feedback loop solution. This hidden flaw worked against his interests, especially as his cancer always tried to game the system.

Put another way: cancer, per se, is a project. And all projects – no matter how small or large, how technical or simple - all projects have embedded feedback loops of which we are all players who receive information, evaluate, transmit and act on that information. Or, maybe some of us don't.

If all we do is report events and act on the directions of others, we forever remain outside the value of our feedback loop. We allow ourselves to become fungible commodities, but which could otherwise be the means by which to improve our job standing, our health and our lives.

In effect: Static information in, static information out.

It was this limited sense of vision and lack of bi-directional engagement that Ping carried forward into how he approached his job and his cancer. Thus, his cancer management, or mis-management, became a reflection of his lack of advocacy for himself, his job and his life. As the cancer advanced it easily did so at the expense of its host, Ping.

So, goals? What goals?

Ping was doing his best to avoid the cancer issue, even at work, but it wasn't working.

A co-worker had emailed Ping the quarterly production data which Ping needed to turn into meaningful information for the upcoming EOQ, End of Quarter, management meetings. But the data was incomplete, like it always was, because there were key data points missing, or different production quantities produced versus what had been forecast to meet demand. Ping always found this part of his job frustrating and just wished it would go away, much like he wished his bladder cancer would just go away, too.

But until he engaged in the source(s) of the problems with the bad production data, that is until he actually determined the causes of the information gaps, the bad data would be perpetually bad data.

This meant his reports would have gaps that management would complain about and customers would complain because their orders also had problems. While Ping's management team was dysfunctional, too, and accepted his flawed EOQ reports, the firm's customers had begun to react with their feet. Over time they began to go elsewhere. So the firm was becoming fungible due to its own dysfunctionality and it was slowly feeling the effects. This happens in cancer for a similar reason.

In effect Ping was part of the problem and not part of the solution. If he would locate the sources of the bad production data his reports would have value and management could take corrective action. He would become a key part of the feedback loop that helped recognize and address the problems affecting customer dissatisfaction. He would have increased his value to his employer, too, making his job much less fungible.

Likewise, re-deploying the same metaphor for his mis-management of the bladder cancer exposes the flaws in the present treatment program. Flaws like failing to get the most effective and newer treatment technologies, failing to be at a cancer hospital where cancer-specific technologies are the norm rather than the exception - such as PET-CT scanners - and seeking out oncologists who are experts in his bladder cancer and who contribute to the body of knowledge, i.e. through thought leadership and publishing of on-point papers.

Thus, over the long term Ping mis-managed his cancer threat much like he mismanaged his job opportunity by going with the flow, however adverse that was to his best interests. Invariability such people usually fail to understand what went wrong, so that they eventually become expendable.

Then, at the last minute as the wheels come off the wagon, they stand confused while blaming others with no viable options and no possibility of a safe harbor.

Pong: Part A: Recall that Pong had just learned from Dr. Black that two small masses had been identified on his lungs in the most recent CT scan. Pong was outwardly grateful and supportive of the plan put forward to treat his latest relapse by Dr. Black, his oncologist, and Dr. Bernstein, the hospital's oncology radiologist. But he was concurrently apprehensive for the larger implication of the relapse. He felt something was not right, but he chose to keep his counsel to himself.

It had become clear to Pong that what had been normal before the onset of his cancer was never going to be seen again. Running background in his head was the realization of what Penn had meant at their previous luncheon about the "new normal" and he was not comfortable with the evolving view.

When Dr. Black contacted the radiologist who had read the latest CT scan the radiologist had closed their conversation with the disclaimer that he was unable to determine from the CT scan if any melanoma had reached Pong's lymph nodes.

"Well, dammit," Pong vexed, "if he didn't know, then who the hell does? Where are the assurances? Are there limits I should be aware of that I'm not aware of? If the wheels begin to come off the wagon will my team know in enough time? After all, I'm the one who brought up the cold that triggered this sequence of events and I'm not the one peering around inside me with that CT scanner."

Pong, for all his engineering competence, was beginning to react like the last person to get the bad news email. Like, "I'm copied on this, but why am I the last to know?"

As a problem solving person he should know better.

Dr. Black had scheduled Pong for eight doses of IL-2 over a period of three days. The IL-2 was also intended to treat the possibility that the melanoma may have spread to Pong's lymph nodes. An insurance policy.

"Maybe it's in my head. Maybe it's not as bad as I thought. Maybe it's not even there anymore. Maybe my immune system was successful in killing the tumors on my lungs and this entire exercise is just a big insurance policy," Pong thought as he was able to rationalize himself back into a fantasy of the previous normal, even if just for the moment.

In fact, the IL-2 treatments really were intended as an insurance policy because neither Dr. Black nor the radiologist could confirm that there was no melanoma in Pong's lymph nodes. So the IL-2 was selected for its ability to stimulate the production of his T-cells that would then – hopefully - identify and help kill any melanoma cells foolish enough to hang-out in his lymph nodes. And this strategy of hit first and ask questions later would work really well if the melanoma, if it existed, would just cooperate in the IL-2's agenda of suicide-by-proxy. After all, it works in about 15% of all metastasized cases. "Statistically, that is."

Either way he knew he would do his best to get through the IL-2 treatments. The IL-2 would be different from the Dacarbazine treatments he had already experienced because for the IL-2 he would be admitted as an in-patient for at least three days, more likely four days.

Having taken the three pre-meds the day before, Pong and his wife drove to the treatment hospital and arrived slightly ahead of the scheduled appointment at 9 AM. Pong had already made sure the entire process would be treated as personal leave, not sick leave, from work. That is, again, hidden from view.

The first step was a standard blood draw followed by an EKG to test heart function. Next, a nurse collected his vital signs data and attached a heart telemetry unit to monitor heart rate and heart rhythm over the course of the IL-2 treatments. Then, a team of two nurses arrived to insert the PICC line into his arm for him to receive the IL-2. Last, was an X-ray of the PICC line to ensure that it had been properly installed and positioned for the IL-2 IV. All this to receive something he really didn't want, but had been told he needed as an insurance hedge.

By then it was noon and Dr. Black had arrived, reviewed the prep-work and signed-off on the orders for Pong so that he could begin receiving his IL-2 treatments at a rate of one IL-2 IV every eight hours. Pong would receive two that day and three each of the next two days. If all went well he might be released on the morning of the fourth day.

But this treatment sequence was different from his out-patient Dacarbazine treatments. Gone were the casual street clothes, the finite treatment times and getting back to his old normal by late afternoon the same day as the treatment. Today he became an in-patient, someone with a bigger medical problem than before.

He had become someone who had traded those casual street clothes for a cold and ill-fitting hospital gown, someone who might be released in the AM of the fourth day, maybe not. Someone who could plan to return to work, but who might not be returning as before. Pong's new normal had arrived wrapped in an ill-fitting hospital gown with some not too pleasant IV's. Still, Pong was determined to keep this ordeal to himself.

With his wife reading magazines next to his bed, Pong [in the ill-fitting hospital gown and wrapped in blankets to stay warm] began to rethink his situation while he awaited the first IL-2 IV, "So, this is what it's like to be on the other side of out-patient as the new in-patient starts getting worse and as the cancer starts getting stronger. What's next?"

Just as his head-game was starting two nurses arrived to start the first IL-2 IV. The IL-2 volume was based on Pong's weight in Kg's and would be pumped into him through a paperback book-sized IV pump over a period of thirty minutes. The pre-meds he had taken the day before were to ward-off routine side effects of chills, nausea and fever.   But there were other side effects that could occur and he would have to experience them first for the nurses to provide medications to counter the then-occurring adverse effects.

"Great," Pong thought quietly while his wife continued her reading, "I actually have to go off the cliff to find out if the floor is one foot below or a hundred feet down. This wasn't anywhere in the fine print, but I really have no other choice, do I?"

Pong was motoring through the IL-2 treatments as a spectator/player, but not as the person calling the shots. He received information about his treatments, his status, his progress, but he otherwise provided nothing back and only hoped to be leaving soon. The opportunity was there to engage, but he made no effort to implement his feedback loop.

The first two IL-2 treatments passed with no noticeable adverse effects.   But by the end of day two, and the fifth IL-2 treatment, Pong was clearly in substantial headache pain for which Dr. Black had prescribed a codeine-based anti-pain medication, most often known as Oxycodone. For all its justifiable bad press it did get the job done. And by the end of the third day, and the eighth IL-2 treatment, Pong was finished with the IL-2 IV's.

But, because the IL-2 had originally been prescribed as an insurance policy against the spread of the melanoma to Pong's lymph nodes, the real questions still remained: had the melanoma spread to the lymph nodes and, if so, had the IL-2 killed the melanoma? Or, more appropriately, had the IL-2 triggered enough of Pong's T-cells to have killed any and all of the melanoma in his lymph nodes?

In truth no one, including Dr. Black, knew the answer to those or any other collateral questions because they did not know if any melanoma actually existed in Pong's lymph nodes. But they could have!!!

Next in the sequence would be the external beam radiation of the two tumor masses on Pong's lungs. Even if the IL-2 was not determined to have killed any melanoma in Pong's lymph nodes, at least it could be determined to have been active against the tumor masses on his lungs. This was because the pre-IL-2 X-ray of the lungs, when compared to the pre-radiation treatment X-ray, showed that the tumors had shrunk, but by only about 10% to 20%. Still, to a patient struggling with metastasized melanoma this can be encouraging news. "Maybe the IL-2 mercenaries will eventually get the job done," he thought.

Part B: The next step in Pong's treatment cycle was the external beam radiation of the two tumor masses on his lungs. Dr. Black had already prepared Pong that the radiation treatments would be nearly painless. Outwardly Dr. Black was 100% correct because Pong could feel nothing of the actual treatments. But that is not to say there were no effects because there were very emotional effects that no one, neither Dr. Black nor Dr. Bernstein, had told him about.

Because the tumor masses were small, approx. 1 cm in diameter x 3mm in depth on each lung, Dr. Bernstein had scheduled Pong for three radiation treatments each week for two weeks, then a follow-up review two weeks after the last radiation treatment. Dr. Bernstein felt this treatment plan would be adequate to resolve Pong's tumors, but he held out the option to apply more radiation if they proved to be resistant.

The first appointment was not actually the start of the radiation treatments. It was to be fitted for a strap over Pong's abdomen to hold him securely to the radiation table, to immobilize him, as the radiation head was rotated and pivoted a short distance over his lungs. Thus, any movement other than normal breathing would mean the radiation beam could be fired at non-tumor tissue. Like shooting at the rat, but hitting the kitchen window.

Returning for each of his plan's radiation treatments, Pong was reminded, as he lay on the cold table, of the silent genocide taking place each time he heard that 'click' sound and a silent and invisible beam of intense radiation was fired at his lungs. Although he could neither feel nor see the radiation beam as it was fired on command by the technicians, as an engineer he fully understood the reality of what was taking place.

He knew that Dr. Bernstein had designed a radiation treatment regimen whereby he would lie strapped into position on that cold table with his custom fitted cold strap and be moved into position under the head of the radiation unit. Then a technician would initiate Dr. Bernstein's pre-programmed sequence of four radiation beams fired at different angles, as the radiation head silently rotated and pivoted over his chest for each tumor. In all eight beams of intense radiation were fired at his lungs on each of the treatment days.

"Jesus, I'm that same in-patient again who has been moved to a cold slab to be targeted in a glorified microwave. What if they get the wrong program, like for someone other than me? What if they miss? What if the unit gets stuck on? What if...? When does this horror movie end?" Pong thought each time he mounted that cold slab of the radiation table, was strapped-in with his personal strap, was slid under the head of the unit and the technicians re-assured him one more time. Then, just as surely as he had those same thoughts at each treatment he also rationalized each time, "Sure has been a project. But [as before] what other choice do I have?"

As he was approaching the end of the treatments Pong began to think more of the future and was hopeful that all this macabre experience would soon be the last of the melanoma and to wonder how Ping and Penn were progressing. And how much he longed for their friendship and for another lunch together.

For all his angst the two weeks of radiation treatments otherwise passed quickly and without further incident. Pong was soon able to put the real life horror experience of the radiation treatments into the past. The next milestone would be the upcoming appointment with Dr. Bernstein.

While he had approached these treatments with his own form of resignation, like Ping, he had missed the opportunity to invest himself in the treatment process. He could have had a better understanding of where he stood vis-à-vis the cancer and his go-fwd options at the end of the treatments. That is, no feed-back loop.

"Let's find out if those melanoma SOB's really were zapped by Dr. Bernstein's microwave. Actually, I should call Ping and Penn for our next lunch together. I need that," Pong thought as he left his last radiation treatment, hoping to never return.

Penn: The expression "life happens" easily applies to our three characters' experiences with their cancers. While Ping was motoring along in his non-denial-denial mode and Pong was looking for the next exit door as soon as his dual treatment sequence had completed, Penn was into a much different regimen with the ZQT targeted therapy treatment for his relapsed NHL sub-type. His past had taught him that denial was fruitless and, by this much time into the cancer experience, his cancer was incurable and the only exit was the one he did not want. Yet, as alien as these were to him, both defined a place he could not afford to go to unless he had already rationalized throwing in the towel. He knew he had come too far to allow himself to knowingly go down that road.

After all, he had accepted that his wife had given-up on him. He regretted, but accepted her parting   But in addition to himself there was his team of Dr. Collins who was always pulling rabbits out of the hat for him, there was Charlie who had made him her wayward adolescent who she was determined to get onto the right dietetic path, there was Suzette as a surrogate for Dr. Collins, and then there was Sari as his cheerleader.

Surprisingly, even when he allowed himself to think about it, there was always Sari. Somehow he knew that if, for some obscure reason, everyone else found jobs on some remote parts of planet Earth that there would always be Sari. Like there had always been Sari, even when she stood-up that first day and asked his name.

So how could he ever let them down by not working as hard as they did? "Not in my DNA," he thought.

They were a big part of his feedback loop as they accepted his journal of symptoms and other events at each treatment, adjusting the ZQT mcg/Kg doses with the goal of getting him to that distant land of "chronic cancer". If he was the rat caught in the cage, at least in their own ways they had made the whole experience tolerable, like at yesterday's ZQT treatment...

Sari had arrived at the hospital early for a special training program and wasn't there to register him, but she would return soon and had made sure Elaine, one of the staff nurses, registered him and collected his vital signs. After about a half hour Sari arrived. In what seemed like no time she had him set-up with an IV and had the hydration fluids flowing. "Back to happy space," Penn thought.

Being early, Penn was the only one in the infusion area. Soon Suzette stopped by and said that Dr. Collins would likely be by at mid-morning to discuss his recent blood tests because they had noticed an anomaly in his flow cytometry.

"Interesting. I feel fine. Wonder what could be the problem," he thought because he did not have an appointment with Dr. Collins that day.

"Is that important?" Penn asked Suzette in surprise.

"Not really. Don't worry. You're not going off the cliff. We watch our patients closely and we're trying to understand why some of your white blood cells are behaving differently from our expectations. Have you been maintaining your journal?"

"Yes. No change. Just as detailed as the day I arrived," Penn said.

"Do you have it with you today?"

"Yes. It's here on my tablet along with another system I developed that shows the data differently."

"Good," Suzette said, "When Dr. Collins arrives Sari will take you to an exam room to look at your journal alongside our flow cytometry data."

"You sure I'm not having a problem, like with the ZQT?"

"Not likely. But I'll leave the solution of the mystery to Dr. Collins," Suzette said in her typically cold stoicism.

Soon after Suzette had left the area Sari arrived with the pre-meds for his ZQT treatment. Another round of Benadryl, the anti-nausea pill and dexamethasone. But today Penn's curiosity had been tweaked by Suzette's conversation, so he had already resolved to have a cup of coffee as soon as Suzette left so to not be drowsy due to the Benadryl. After all, Penn knew from the original CHOP series how to play his hand with Benadryl.

Just as he was finishing the coffee Sari arrived again to say that Dr. Collins had arrived.

Arriving at the exam room Dr. Collins asked Sari to remain, then Dr. Collins began, "We routinely run pre-treatment analysis on our patients that can include a flow cytometry of their blood. While this is not a requirement for your ZQT treatments, it helps us develop an understanding of how our patients are progressing and to possibly see small problems before they become big obstacles.

We've been doing this for you over the past few treatments and we noticed a change in some of your white blood cells. I have some ideas about what is causing this to occur. First, I want to look at your journal with you to try to correlate the flow cytometry results against the history you've been recording. Can we look at the journal?" Dr. Collins asked.

"Sure. But as I explained to Suzette, there's the journal and there's another system I created that shows the journal data differently. You may want to see both," Penn said as he started-up his tablet computer.

"So," Penn began, "this is my medical history journal. It's organized with each event logged to a specific date. And [pointing to the individual entries in the journal] these are all the events as they've been recorded whether at this hospital or elsewhere. As you can see, there's plenty of detail but not for the sake of being too detailed.

In the other system the data from the journal has been transformed. This makes it easy to see treatments and events that might otherwise not be visible by just looking at the journal entries. Think of it like you might a financial statement."

"That's very interesting," Dr. Collins said. "No one else has done this as a patient. I can see each of your ZQT treatments in the Journal and then in the other system. As I compare our flow cytometry results to your graph of the entries an interesting pattern emerges.

During the post-ZQT treatment period of up to two to three days you have almost none of the classic symptoms, but your T-cells have greatly increased. On the other hand, looking back to when you originally arrived here following your P-3 clinical trial the same pattern did not occur. Your immune system was not producing T-cells in the volumes it is producing them today.

This is an important finding and it may point to a new level of progress you are making against your NHL cancer. In other words, the difficulty you had with the ZQT at the outset appears to be in the past and your immune system now appears to be producing T cells even in the presence of the ZQT treatment."

Penn saw the opportunity and quickly asked, "Does this mean I am reaching a state of being cured?"

"No, that's not where this conversation is headed. Nor is it a possibility for your cancer.

I am increasingly of the opinion that your immune system has learned to tolerate the ZQT and is now playing an upgraded support role with the production of the new T-cells.

Today there is no cure for your sub-type of NHL. Sorry, that's just the hard reality. But looked at from the positive, the ZQT is doing a good job of attacking your cancer cells as soon as you get the IV and your immune system is now able to respond as it should by producing a greater quantity of white blood cells just when they are needed after the ZQT infusion.

Unfortunately those T-cells do not continue to be produced in sufficient volumes by your immune system and by the time you return for the next ZQT treatment you have become deficient. Do you see why it's not likely you will ever be cured of this cancer?" Dr. Collins said.

"I think I'm beginning to understand," Penn replied.

"In reality it's the detail you are maintaining in your journal and the other system that we do not collect because it occurs after you have left the hospital. It appears to confirm our conclusions. Sure wish other patients could do the same.

I don't see you getting off the ZQT treatments. Not at all. Rather, I would not be surprised to one day see you transition to a maintenance plan that includes ZQT as your primary treatment. Compared to the situation you were in when you first became a patient here you've come a very long way.

Your cancer is rare and incurable. I almost never see a future past 18 to 24 months for patients with this sub-type of NHL.

Almost never. But you seem to be reversing that pattern. Congratulations."

"Actually the thanks go to you and to Sari and my team here, not to me. It appears that the journal and the other system were a help?" Penn asked.

"Absolutely, because they were able to confirm the conclusions we had been making about your post-ZQT treatments that we were unable to see otherwise. These are key parts of your feedback loop that takes the guess work out of the test results we're seeing.

Without them we would be wandering in the desert unable to confirm our conclusions. And they form a valuable link to the future because we can revise our opinions as you get ZQT treatments and you make post-treatment entries in the journal. Do they take a lot of time to maintain?" Dr. Collins asked.

"Actually, very little. It takes so little time that they're a simple habit to maintain as current. Maybe five minutes a day."

"Only five minutes. That's amazing. Even if we are wrong, and I don't believe we are wrong, it is a valuable way for us to synch your treatments and flow cytometry history against your actual post-treatment experiences.

Let's do this again in the future to see if you really are on track to a maintenance plan. I am beginning to think you are and this is a huge difference from what I routinely see in others.

Sari will see you back to your IV chair. I think you'll soon be feeling the effects of the Benadryl. Thanks Penn. This was very helpful and it will be useful for my other patients who are also on ZQT," Dr. Collins said as they left the exam room together.

Dr. Collins could see the Benadryl was beginning to overcome the coffee's caffeine. Soon Sari had him back in his IV chair and Penn was quickly asleep.

While he slept, Sari and another nurse arrived to check Penn's Id and start the ZQT IV.

Waking about fifteen minutes before the ZQT IV finished, Penn had a few moments of quiet to himself to reflect on the conversation with Dr. Collins and against his condition eighteen months ago. "If I hadn't lived it myself, I wouldn't believe it. I'm caught in my own feed-back loop," he thought in quiet reflection.

"Do you just come here to nap?" Sari said softly as she approached his chair to detach the IV line.

"Hadn't thought of it that way, but do you take-in overnighters? I'm solo now and it would shorten my commute."

"Right. Next you'll expect a meal plan. And you'll especially want your café mocha to be catered. You tourist patients are all the same," she said without ever looking at him while she placed a bandage over the wound where the IV line had been on his arm.

"Not my idea, but I like it. Actually, I think I'll try some variety and do lunch in the *Atrium*," Penn said in quick retort.

"Suit yourself, but actually we send the leftovers to the *Atrium* café for those not lucky enough to have lunch up here in patient-ville. Have it your way. See you same time next week?" she said with a gentle hand to his back as they walked past the nurses' station.

Undeterred even by Sari, and it being nearly 1 PM, Penn was determined to unwind the remaining tiredness of the Benadryl over a café mocha and a Caesar salad in the *Atrium*.

The "*Atrium*" was neither a café nor a restaurant. It was a naturally lit, large indoor courtyard accessible from any point on the compass with potted fig trees, a high skylight, not-uncomfortable café-style tables and chairs and a center of the atrium fountain that provided just the right amount of distraction and background white noise for casual or intimate conversations. In effect, the setting had been well conceived for this hospital's unique clientele.

After ordering his café mocha and a Caesar salad in the adjacent bistro, Penn located a table off the main traffic areas and away from the noise of the fountain, but still with excellent views of the fountain's displays and the passersby. He was nearly finished with the salad when he heard two familiar voices approaching from behind.

"Did you think you could have this entire view all to yourself?" was Charlie's un-subtle interrogation as she approached with Sari.

"What a pleasant surprise. Please join me," Penn said, re-composed for the moment.

"OK, but only to inspect and pass judgment on what you're having for lunch. Hmmm, I see you are having one of those café mochas Sari has told me you have a fetish for and is that a Caesar salad that has a dressing with both calories and carbs?" was Charlie's opening dietetic-centric salvo.

"Charlie, the café mocha is my reward for abstinence and the Caesar salad is the most benign entré I could find. I would offer you some of the café mocha, but I know you would decline in envy," Penn said with a smile to lob the ball back into Charlie's court while Sari remained silent.

Just then Charlie's cell phone rang. She looked at the code and quickly said, "A patient I've been expecting just arrived. Sari, please watch Penn and do your best to protect him from himself. Sorry, but I've gotta run. Bye," as she disappeared beyond the fountain.

"I didn't mean to ruin your lunch, we just ...," Sari started to say.

"Sari, I'm delighted you stopped-by. But please look over to the left of the fountain ... into the corridor. Am I right? Is that Mimi with her husband? She looks so frail and weak," Penn said in a voice of disbelief.

"Yes. It is Mimi. She means a lot to you doesn't she?"

"It pains me deeply to see her struggle that way. I need to go over...?"

But as Penn started to move Sari placed her hand firmly on his arm that was still on the table, "Penn ... It's best for both of you that you don't," while a gentle, but in-control look formed on Sari's face and in her voice.

"Sari, what's going-on? I thought she was ...?" Penn said as he moved closer to emotional shock while slowly sitting back into his chair.

"Have you finished your salad?" Sari said as she gently began to edge the conversation into shallower waters.

"Yes, I guess you're right, but I just ..."

"I have to get back to my other patients. Let's walk over to the garage elevators," Sari said.

Walking slowly across the *Atrium* to the elevators in the opposite direction from where Mimi had gone Sari began, "Penn please listen to me. I know where you are right now and I deeply feel your pain in a way you may not be able to understand, but please trust me. Please do that for me. Please?"

"OK. I'll try," he said emotionally troubled.

"Both of you are my patients and I know how much you mean to each other and I wish I could make these words be different. I wish so much that I could make your pain go away, but I feel I must share something with you in confidence. OK?

Penn please look at me … [as Penn adjusts his gaze into Sari's eyes as his fill with tears and her hands held his firmly] …

Please place your trust in me … Do you remember what I told you about the GVHD problem Mimi was having after her stem cell transplant? [Penn nodded yes, but with emotional pain in his face]. Penn you may need to prepare yourself for some very difficult news, not tomorrow or the next day, but soon. Maybe a few weeks at most.

Do you understand?" Sari said as she held Penn's hands and could feel his grip grow tighter.

"No, Sari, I guess I just don't get it. And maybe I never will. Maybe I've been so heads down and into me that I'm just not any good at the reality of losing friends, especially those who've meant so much to me and who've helped make it possible for me to be here. I'm probably not making much sense. I'm sorry for being so weak-kneed right now."

"I know this news is a lousy way to start the weekend, but do us both a big favor. Send Mimi another "Thinking of you" card and sign it 'Penn and a Friend'. Don't forget that I'm in this with both of you. Can you do that for us? Please?"

Still looking at her, "OK, yes, I'll do it. At least you've given me a mission. Thanks," Penn said as he backed into the elevator and offered a feeble wave good-bye. But the emotional stress in his face said it all.

But before the elevator doors could close Sari placed her hand between the doors to take one more risky step, "Don't forget you have to be back here next Wednesday AM. Be here early. OK?"

"OK. Another mission. Will do."

WIFM - Reality Assessment #9

Because to not do is to fail.

Ping: *Regrettably, Ping is fungible in his job and the job reflects his value to himself, i.e. he plays out the mis-management of his cancer with the same dysfunctional practices he pursues in his job.*

At work Ping could increase his job's value to his employer by simply ferreting-out the causes of the defective production data which would help in the retention of existing customers. Likewise, in his cancer situation he could add value to himself by advocating for oncologists who specialize in bladder cancer and who are affiliated with a recognized cancer-centric hospital.

Instead he takes the path of least resistance, or the path of lowest apparent cost, or any path that does not require him to engage in the process of finding answers to challenging and unpleasant problems. This is more denial for denial's sake. The result is that he is outside his own cancer feed-back loop.

It's avoidance of responsibility that leads directly to systemic failure where and when it will incur the greatest loss and pain.

Pong: Pong, on the other hand, has already raised the critical questions again and again and he knows the costs. He knows his doctors should be finding the answers and he knows he is the one most at risk. But, even as he acknowledges these threshold truths, he avers in taking the next steps.

Cancer does not suffer those of us who fail to take the offense, or who abdicate our responsibilities or who fail to add value. Left to its own agenda cancer will add value to itself at the expense of its host because cancer never sleeps.

Late in the game Pong began to reflect on the transition that is underway as he considers the consequences of having become an in-patient versus the less rigorous experiences when he was just an out-patient. His cancer wasn't sleeping then, it's not sleeping now.

Metastasized melanoma is a very serious life threat. Will his relapsed melanoma really be brought under control with an "insurance policy" oriented treatment regimen, which his subconscious already questions? Like Ping, Pong is dis-engaged from his feed-back loop when it could be most valuable to him.

And, for what? His unwillingness/avoidance to take the next steps to insist on answers to which he already has the questions!

Penn: Unlike either Ping or Pong, who are mirroring each other, Penn has sought ways to add value because he wants to regain his health. Also, by knitting himself into a pro-active support team at a comprehensive cancer hospital he has evolved a sense of mutual responsibility whereby the contributions of Penn and his team members add value even while his cancer never sleeps.

Penn's efforts to apply his own creativity actually add value to his team's ability to draw conclusions not otherwise available to the team. And, it adds value in how Dr. Collins approaches the treatment of others. These simple efforts expanded Dr. Collins' concept of the possible against the stark historic experience. This created extensible value-add. Nothing fungible or characteristic of avoidance here. **Totally offense, not defense.**

And yet there will be those times when all we can do is our best to save ourselves. Those times can be very painful experiences as we are powerless to help others with cancer, even those who have been so helpful to us. Incredibly, there will be pain that exceeds even the pain from our cancer.

Penn is extremely fortunate to be at a recognized cancer-centric hospital with such a broad and deep team.

BP Score Card:
Ping = 0, Pong = 0, Penn = 1 - Always be engaging your cancer feed-back loop.

#10 Staying In-touch:
The Next Luncheon of Ping, Pong & Penn

I can't believe it.

Even before he had met with his oncologist to review the results of the most recent treatments, Pong had already followed-up on his plan to schedule the next luncheon with Ping and Penn. He was looking forward to returning to *Café Soleil* with his friends, much like we re-acclimate to liking our ruts when we're facing adversity.

Pong knew Ping. He knew how Ping was likely to be at lunch with him and Penn. Ping would be an active follower and could be counted on to still be a true believer in his team, even though others were beginning to see through his myopia and how it was disserving him. Pong, on the other hand, was beginning to think he needed a newer perspective.

Hoping that his timing wasn't too late, Pong was optimistic that this lunch with Penn might provide some new insight into his own cancer predicament. While it was unlikely Ping could provide that insight, Penn was a different matter.

Pong knew Penn had a very challenging cancer situation and had had to endure multiple treatment regimens for his cancer. Maybe, just maybe, his friend would have some ideas he would share over a casual conversation at lunch. After all, his own treatment program was showing signs of strain and he was beginning to think he needed some fresh thinking. His transition from out-patient to in-patient was certainly the latest validation of that concern.

While Pong was not even close to considering radical surgery to his own melanoma treatment program, it was obvious that he teetered somewhere between Ping, who was not making progress, and Penn who appeared to be making progress.

Pong knew his own slippage confirmed that he needed to re-think a new dialogue. He was hopeful the lunch with Penn would provide that opportunity.

As with the previous lunch, Pong had already decided to arrive early. If Penn arrived early, too, it would be his best chance to get the conversation going in the right direction without Ping's own well intentioned vectoring. It was certainly better than getting trapped into another chit-chat conversation about the ladies in the park.

Being an engineer, punctuality had been inscribed into Pong's DNA at birth. From that time onward he was just following the script. So for the 12 Noon lunch Pong arrived at 11:45. He parked his Honda in a space on the opposite side of the park and walked the fifty-or-so yards through the park to the front steps of *Café Soleil*.

For a moment he stood with one foot on the lowest step looking back across the park through the pines. He knew he would see Ping's SUV before Ping saw him, but he did not know what Penn would be driving. Simple as it might be, he was quietly hoping his plan would pan-out.

"You appear to be lost. Do you need directions?" was the familiar voice from just a few yards behind him. His heart leaped a small bound because he knew that voice to be Penn's. The plan had worked!

"Well, maybe I am, lost that is. Great to see you. Glad you could be here today," Pong said clearly pleased that Penn had arrived so soon.

"Wouldn't have missed it for the world. I've been in a funk these past few days and your call brightened my horizon. How have you been?" Penn asked.

"Everyone is well at home and the job is doing well, too. Keeps me off the streets. I see Ping just drove-up on the other side of the park. Let's go get a table on the terrace," Pong said to make sure he kept his agenda headed in his intended direction before Ping joined them.

Pong had previously reserved a table overlooking the park and underneath a red awning with a propane heater. Having just sat down Pong asked casually, "If you don't mind me asking, are you still with the same oncologist you told us about last time we met?"

"Interesting question. If I recall our previous lunch I had already emerged from the CHOP treatments and I probably had very little hair at that time. So the answer would be 'No'. I've moved on. Why do you ask?" Penn replied as Ping was then walking up the stairs to the terrace.

"Ping, good to see you again. You're looking great," Penn said while reaching to shake hands as Ping approached their table.

"I saw Pong's Honda, so I parked in the next space. But I didn't know what you would be driving," Ping said to Penn as he sat down at their table.

"Well there have been a few changes in my life. It's been up, then down, then up and I decided to do something to shorten the downs. My Volvo wagon had a lot of miles and it wasn't worth much, but it still ran well. I decided to keep the Volvo and to get a sports car for those times when I need to shorten my downs. So I bought a Porsche," Penn confessed with pride to his friends.

"So, Penn, any chance you need a driver during your down spells?" Ping responded.

"Gee, thanks Ping."

"Does it have a sunroof so you can let the sunshine in and the bad vibes out," Pong inquired.

"Well, no. It's a cabriolet so the bad vibes just get vaporized as the sunshine pours in all over," Penn said with a smile.

"911?" Pong asked while looking at the menu.

"Yes. In fact it's just behind you by only half a block. It's black with a red leather interior," Penn said.

As they finished ordering their meals Ping asked, "Second childhood?"

"Maybe, but there's more to it than that. My life had become a kluge and I felt that I needed a way to escape reality now and then. Midway through one of my chemo treatments my wife served notice that she felt she needed a break. It's a long story, but she now lives in Charleston near her sister and we communicate infrequently via email. I guess it's a reality of cancer that other's lives change, too."

"Actually I've wondered about that same experience from time to time, but it seems that every time it's running as a background thought my wife comes through as my biggest cheerleader," Ping said in reaction.

"I've been through lots of different chemo treatments, even though I am still on her health insurance plan. Seams crazy doesn't it?" Penn added as their meals arrived.

"After crisscrossing the country, doctor after doctor, hospital after hospital, and plan after plan etc, etc I am now in a non-chemo-chemo treatment at a major cancer center that is right here in our back yard. Imagine, in our own back yard and I missed that at the outset because I wasn't being my own advocate."

"Sounds like you've been through several remission-relapse cycles," Pong asked following his original agenda.

"That's right, Pong. By the time I entered my current hospital and treatment plan there had been four separate plans followed by four relapses of those plans. What was common was that the remissions just became shorter and shorter. The last one was only about three weeks long, maybe none if I am totally honest."

"Even though I've had far fewer relapses the time intervals have not really shortened, so I guess I'm still ahead in that area," Ping said.

"Each shorter relapse must be unsettling? Pong asked.

"You're right on that one, Pong. I was a true believer when I got that cell call from my first oncologist that I was 'cancer free'. Then, three relapses later, I came face-to-face with the reality of nearly zero time of remission. Zero is a very steep cliff. That was a very unnerving experience."

"How did you handle the problem?" Ping asked, looking at the Porsche.

"It was very difficult OJT at first, but I realized that the cancer was not going away – took a long time for that light bulb to click-on for me – so I set the goal of reaching a state of cancer as a chronic condition and to do so I had to become my own advocate. Then, as each challenge emerged I learned to maintain three lists of options on a 3x5 index card. One list was of oncologists who specialized in my sub-type of non-Hodgkin's Lymphoma, the second and third were of two types of potential treatments for my cancer. I still carry it with me. Here it is [as Penn pulled the folded card from his wallet]."

As the waiter cleared the table of their dishes Pong realized he had achieved his objective for the get together and said reflectively while still looking at Penn's card, "Sure wish we could have had this conversation earlier."

On that note Penn added, "Well, I'm not out of the woods yet and may never be free of the cancer. But I now see each challenge differently. With a goal of my cancer as a chronic condition, one that is still incurable but possibly manageable. And I see each of cancer's challenges as speed bumps that have to be solved incrementally to achieve that goal of chronic cancer. That's where my own cancer advocacy comes in. It's up to me to make this happen."

"But isn't that really the job of your medical team?" Ping asked.

"Yes, it is to the extent it fits within their skillset. After all it is my life that's at risk, so I believe it's my responsibility to bear my share of the burden. Maybe that's part of the reason why there are so many deceased cancer patients elsewhere."

"OK, I see your point. Hadn't thought of it that way, but maybe I should," Pong said in reflection.

"And the Porsche has a role here, too?" Ping asked rhetorically.

"It does. I have an incurable cancer, an incredible oncologist, a pretty nurse, no wife to speak of and I don't even have a dog. So every now and then I need a way to try to make sense of all the confusion. Hence, the Porsche. Hope I'm not sounding like I've had too much wine."

"Are you saying you think you need a dog, too, when you have a beautiful Porsche?" Pong was quick to react.

"Thanks Pong [Penn said with a smile], I needed that. But, yes. I've been thinking of getting a friend, like a wire fox terrier. What I call a 'WFT'. He could ride shotgun in the Porsche. Any ideas?"

"Hell, I'll ride shotgun and I don't bark," Ping said.

"Back to something you just said, about having been through lots of chemo treatments. What has changed?" Ping asked, which surprised Pong.

"After our last get together I was in a 'Watch and See' kind of plan with my second oncologist. That failed after a few months. He then created a home brewed non-clinical-clinical trial. That was a disaster, too. With him my treatments had become a high risk crap-shoot.

Using my list I then located a very bright oncologist at a distant cancer hospital, but there were logistical problems and, well, it was a non-starter. So next on my list I located an oncologist who was not as far away and who had several clinical trials in open enrollment. I enrolled in one of his clinical trials, but it failed too. By the end of that clinical trial I had failed four separate plans, but each with greater severity and increasingly shorter remissions.

I still wasn't ready to throw in the towel. Nor had I become a non-believer, but I did think I needed some new thinking if my chances of survival were to improve.

I've learned the hard truths of cancer. It never sleeps and when it returns it does so with a vengeance as it learns and adapts.

I had been updating my list of options by oncologists who specialized in my flavor of non-Hodgkin's lymphoma and various chemos for my cancer. Turns-out there was an oncologist specializing in my rare sub-type of non-Hodgkin's lymphoma very close to where we are sitting right now. Had I been smart enough to have created that list of options at the outset I might still have a wife, but not likely the Porsche."

"An interesting problem," Ping responded.

"Well, there's more to it than my off-hand remark may suggest. My current oncologist is a specialist in my very rare cancer. I've learned that those specialists are only to be found where cutting edge research is being done, not out in rural hospitals, or even their affiliates. So if you find that you have cancer your interests are probably best served by making your way to a recognized cancer-centric hospital. That's where there are oncologists who routinely treat your type of cancer and where research and clinical trials are always underway. You have too much at stake to do otherwise."

"Are you still there?" Pong asked.

"I am. Yes, and still with the same oncologist and the same primary nurse. I may transition to a maintenance treatment plan in the future, if I continue to make progress. But I am no longer queued-up on death's door step,"

"Let me add this up: you have a great oncologist who specializes in your rare cancer and who has brought you back from the edge of the cliff, you have a drop dead gorgeous black Porsche cabriolet and you have a pretty nurse. Why are you thinking of getting a wire fox terrier?" Ping inquired.

"It's a long story, but suffice it to say that my nurse thinks I need a friend,"

"Pong, I think Penn needs a shrink, not a fuzzy four-legged friend," Ping said rhetorically.

"I'm pondering that one too," Pong said following Ping.

"Penn, in my opinion you need to return to reality. Just loan me your Porsche and you can take my SUV for your journey back to reality," Ping said in jest.

"Thanks, Ping. I'll give it some thought."

"But, seriously, that's an incredible journey," Pong said next.

"Looking back on it, you're right. At the time I needed a plan, so I set a goal. The reality was that I had, and still have, a rare and aggressive cancer so I decided to accept it as permanent and to strive to achieve a state of cancer as a chronic condition. Next, I resolved to become my own advocate. Admittedly I had some learning to do. It was a challenge, but I did it. Truthfully, anyone can do what I did if they are willing to believe in themselves. When I first met Dr. Collins, my current oncologist, I just knew in my heart that everything I had been through had paid-off. The same can be said for Sari, my nurse. They are the ones who've made all my progress possible."

"Her name really is Sari?" Ping asked.

"Yes. Her parents were from Holland and Israel. They moved here when she was quite young. But both her parents are deceased now."

"Married? Kids? Dog?" Ping asked again.

"No. None. Doesn't know I have the Porsche, either. Just thinks I need a local support team. Hence the dog," Penn replied matter-of-factly.

"And she wants you to get a wire fox terrier, what she calls a 'WFT'. Got it. I rest my case," Ping said.

"This has been another great lunch and we should get together more often. But one more question that is not about your struggles with the Porsche or the pretty nurse-thing. And I can't believe her name is actually Sari. You said your cancer is aggressive and incurable, but you may transition to a maintenance plan, right?" Pong asked in guarded disbelief.

"Yes. Unlike any of my previous doctors Dr. Collins actually took on my case as a challenge. And Sari was a key member of the team from the outset. That's because all patients are part of a team at this cancer hospital, and so are the other doctors and nurses and PA's also part of its on-going patient-focused teams.

In that sense I am a project and my team members are evaluated internally by the hospital's management on how they are able to return their patients to good health. So no patient is just another customer. The result of being in their care is that what had not been possible at the other hospitals, this team and hospital have achieved as though it's standard operating procedure for them. Does that make sense?"

"Incredible," Pong said.

"In a way, it is. At this cancer hospital what I've just told you is only a piece of the larger picture. The entire hospital is a single entity that operates around the concept of multi-disciplinary treatment of its patients. So my 'chronic cancer' and my 'cancer advocacy' concepts synch-up perfectly.

In effect I am as much a part of my team as are all of the others on my team. If Dr. Collins thinks I am entering a risk area for cardiology, just by example, the hospital's multi-disciplinary team will already have reviewed my file with Dr. Collins before one of the cardiologists contacts me for an appointment. Not the other way around, or worse. Like finding out too late there had been a cardiology problem.

Otherwise the hospital could lose a patient after it had already made a substantial investment, even though the resources had existed all along to have prevented that failure. You just can't get this kind of coverage outside of such a dedicated cancer care hospital."

"Thanks. You've really answered my questions," Pong said.

"Well, maybe Pong's grateful but I'm still envious. I mean, you obviously have a great oncologist, your cancer condition is improving, there's the Porsche cabriolet-thing and you have a pretty nurse, too. Where do I enroll?" Ping said to add some levity.

"Both of you are great friends. Even if it is cancer that brought us together, I am very grateful. Let's do this again toward the end of summer while it's still warm enough to sit out on the terrace like today," Penn said knowing his contribution had made a difference and feeling good about being part of the threesome.

The luncheon also lifted his spirits from his concerns for Mimi.

"I like that idea," Pong said to make sure it had his buy-in.

"Me too," Ping said, "but, I'll be looking for an update on your progress under the duress of the Porsche and the WFT. And make sure you carry lots of sun block," Ping added as they parted.

WIFM - Reality Assessment #10

And, that is why you will fail.

Ping: *He really is along for the ride, at least until the next relapse happens. Then, he'll react like it can't be true. Like, "Where did that come from?"*

Even as he heard Penn base his progress on the twin "DNA-like Framework" of his cancer advocacy and on striving to reach a condition of chronic cancer against such a determined adversary, Ping never saw the fit-ability to himself. It's little wonder that there are no supportive base-pairs forming to support him.

Pong: *After this much time, all of his treatments, becoming an in-patient where he had been an out-patient and his melanoma having metastasized, Pong is finally reviewing his to-date progress and opening-up to new ideas. But will it turn into action?*

He has the incentive when he says earlier, "I've become an in-patient where I was once just an out-patient and I just don't want to believe it could be happening to me. Just don't want to do it." And he went to the lunch with Ping and Penn with an agenda to inquire about how Penn had progressed so far.

Penn has literally provided Pong and Ping - you too - a road map. He has spelled-out a vision, a determination to prevail and he has shown that it is possible to be successful, even in cancer, if we are just willing to believe in ourselves and take pragmatic, make-sense, steps.

Like: set a goal of chronic cancer, become your own advocate, create and maintain a list of oncologists and treatments, don't take any wooden nickels. And always be on the offense.

But we've been here before with Pong. Now that he has Penn's road map and he sees the problems in his own treatments, will he act while he still has time to do so?

Penn: *Today's luncheon is quite a turnaround for Penn from when we first met him in "Cancer: Who Gave Me Cancer?"*

He is supported by the twin strands of his "DNA-like framework" of cancer as a chronic condition and his own cancer advocacy. He has formed multiple base-pairs that link his "DNA-like framework." He has a list of oncologists and available treatments, he has learned to believe in himself as he builds more base-pairs to strengthen his "My Chronic Cancer" and his "My Cancer Advocacy" helical strands!

In brief, at this point in the cancer experience Penn still has the most threatening cancer, although Pong's melanoma holds high risks. But he is prepared with a very pro-active team at a comprehensive cancer hospital and he is improving measurably.

Only Penn is changing certainty. That is why he will not fail. Isn't that what it's all about?

BP Score Card:
Ping = 0, Pong = 1, Penn = 0 - Cancer is such a crushing black hole, we need to always be open to new ideas.

#11 On Losing Friends to Cancer

In the deepest sorrow of my life I could only say goodbye.

Penn: Did you send Mimi that card? Are you OK now?," Sari began her usual pre-treatment interrogation in that soft accent as she greeted Penn a few minutes earlier than his normal arrival time in the reception area.

Looking at Sari as though he was missing the last 24 hours of sleep, which was mostly true, Penn said softly, "I'm as OK as it's possible to be, I guess. I found a really nice card for Mimi and signed it 'Penn and a Friend'. Like she couldn't figure-out that one. I spent the entire weekend thinking about only two things."

"Maybe she will be OK. Maybe you just saw her at her lowest and she'll turn it around. Maybe I was too candid ... I'm really sorry for what I said," Sari confided defensively in the otherwise vacant reception area.

"Sari, you said what needed to be said in your most compassionate and honest way. And hopefully all the dark clouds will just blow away. I sincerely hope you'll be right. But I guess I needed you to be in-touch with me as only you could be. Lately, seems like as much as I want to be moving-on I'm just not able to move at all. A real change for me.   Thanks for being here so early this morning," Penn said in a low voice of painful reflection.

"Would a hug help?"

"No one has said that to me in a long time [as they embraced],"

"Well ... Let's get you started on your hydration and I want to talk to you about something else ... about your treatments that is," Sari said as she dropped her right hand to the small of his back to start them walking into the infusion area.

With Sari's ever efficient presence Penn's ZQT treatment went as all his previous treatments had gone - perfect. But today there was no Charlie to keep him on her straight and narrow diet regimen.

And Dr. Collins was off-site at a conference, but Suzette did stop-by to the let Penn and Sari know his blood results were normal and she had signed the orders for his ZQT treatment.

Even his Benadryl induced nap came and went without a hitch. He had long-since become accustomed to leaving his wrist with the Id band exposed as he napped so Sari and another nurse could read it to start the ZQT treatment sequence without waking him.

Just as he was waking, Sari arrived to detach the remaining hydration bag and remove the IV from his left arm.

"At least when you're in a slump this place can be counted on to have its act together," Penn thought reflectively.

"We didn't get a chance to talk about this earlier, but you should be thinking more about getting a port installed. I know you're probably going to say 'No' and give me more push-back, but it's getting much harder to insert the IV into your vein each time we give you a ZQT treatment, or even just for a routine blood draw. I am really bringing it up for your own benefit. So, before you say 'No', again, just give it some thought and we can discuss it next time. OK?"

With his defenses already lowered and the sleep from the Benadryl still ebbing from within to her surprise to he said, "OK, I'll think it over."

"You sure you're OK to drive home?" Sari, asked as she placed a bandage over the IV insertion wound on his arm.

"Nothing a café mocha won't fix in about fifteen minutes."

"Why am I not surprised?" she said in exasperation. "Be here early next time and we can talk about the port-thing. OK?"

"Sure, but any update news about Mimi?"

"Nothing yet, but we'll talk about it next time if you can be here early," she said as they walked to the exit together.

For Penn the following week just plain dragged from one day to the next. It was another of those weeks of rest to allow his organs, especially his liver, to recover from the stresses of the ZQT treatments.

With no wife at home he felt aimless. He was finding there were even limits to how often it was possible to escape reality, even in a Porsche cabriolet.

Every now and then he found himself thinking that maybe Sari did have a point that he needed that wire fox terrier, what Ping had called a "fuzzy four-legged friend". But for now, Penn concluded, the Porsche was the limit of his commitment to escapism. Besides, he reasoned, if he started conceding even little things like a WFT to Sari there may be no end in sight.

With no one else at home the solitude had assumed a new dimension. Even when nothing else was happening, no phone calls, no friends stopping-by, still there was something else going on inside his head.

Work had lost its magic, too. It no longer held his attention like it had in the past. Things like the pursuit of business goals were losing their luster and he had to admit to himself that he was beginning to question the value of what he was currently doing in his job. Even to questioning what he had been doing in his job for so many years.

Sure I need to work to earn a living, but is this it? If I only have one ticket in life is this how I want to spend it? If not this, then what?" It seemed that one question begot two more questions, but none with answers.

What Ping had said at *Café Soleil* kept ringing in his head, like a song on perpetual repeat, over and over, "it seems that every time it's running as a background thought my wife comes through as my biggest cheerleader".

"Did my cancer really change her so much that she stopped being my cheerleader? Gee, maybe we just thought we were each other's cheerleader. Maybe we weren't.

Was it just an illusion from the start? Life's so short and precious. Imagine spending an entire life with someone only to find out over a disease like cancer, like when the chips are really down, that there really never was anything to the relationship. Like she never was my cheerleader!

Even after our lunch I still don't know where Ping is with his cancer. But he sure has the world with a fence around it when it comes to his wife. After all they've been through together she's still his 'biggest cheerleader'. Cancer or no cancer, how lucky is he for her!"

As the morning of his next treatment arrived Penn was no better off than when he had last left the hospital. But his next ZQT treatment lay directly across his path and even it was a welcome break from the relentless thoughts and answerless questions. Truly something familiar to look forward to get away from that broken head game that would not end.

With the haunting beauty of Andrea Bocelli and Sarah Brightman's song "*Time to Say Goodbye*" just ending on the Porsche's radio and Sari's last words still tugging at him, Penn parked the car in the hospital's garage, had his parking ticket stamped and headed up to the second floor and into the same reception area where it had all begun at this cancer hospital only about two years ago.

Even if he really was making grudging progress against his incurable cancer this treatment just felt different. Subconsciously he knew the threat was still there, a threat that no amount of Porsche drives could erase. With that tune still on repeat in his head and the echo of Sari's last words still clear about being here early, where was Mimi?

Then, off the elevator with one right turn followed by a left into the reception area and - there was Sari, alone and staring up through the misted-over skylights.

This was not in the script. He knew he was supposed to arrive first and wait and wait and, but there she was. Beautiful, but lost. And why so early?

"Hi, I …," Penn began.

"I was hoping you would be here early. Is it OK … I mean can we…?" she struggled to say.

"I didn't expect to see you so early. I couldn't sleep at all last night. Since we're both here, can I talk you into a café mocha in the *Atrium* so neither of us falls asleep too early?" Penn said jumping in to head off her inability to finish her own sentence.

"Uh, yes. Yes, you're right. Mocha would be better than a Benadryl right now. But … I'm in scrubs, so no cash. Can you….?" She said, still fumbling her words out of character.

"Haven't bought that WFT yet, so I still have some cash. We can do it."

A half smile of thanks from Sari, as her eyes gave an approving OK.

After a wordless elevator ride to the *Atrium* Penn said, "I'll get us a couple of café mochas. Be right back."

Their café table was tucked under a tall, potted fig tree just far enough from the fountain's display to still carry on a conversation, but not be overheard. Penn set the mochas on the table and looked into Sari's very red azure eyes.

"Are you going to tell me what I think you're here to tell me, but it's hurting you as much as it's now hurting me?" he said in a troubled voice just above the sound of the fountain's falling water, while looking into her beautiful but swollen eyes.

"It was pneumonia from the GVHD. It happened yesterday. She went peacefully. No pain. I could see it coming. I made sure I was her head nurse so I could be with her in those final hours. Pulled a few strings. She just slept away with no pain. I'm glad I was her nurse, but I'm so sad. I'm so sorry to be such a wreck. It's not supposed to happen this way. Not in my script," she said as quiet tears made dark wet circles on her indigo blue scrubs.

"Maybe I should have been somewhere else, but I wanted to be there with her and her family. [Lots of quiet tears while looking askance to the fountain.] Can't tell you why, but I just had to be there."

Reaching across their table, Penn gently blotted her tears with a tissue while covering her hand that lay limp on the table.

"I owe you an apology that I didn't call, but I didn't call because I knew how much Mimi meant to you and down deep I just believed you needed to remember her as that beautiful lady, so full of life, the one you loved in your own way and who helped you get to where you are today. Can you forgive me for not calling?" Sari said quietly through a steady stream of tears.

"Sari, there's nothing to forgive. This past week of rest - what a ridiculous term - was one of the most stressful weeks of my life. Something, can't describe what it was, but something kept running background till finally this morning on the drive to the hospital I just knew it had to be about Mimi and it wasn't going to be good. I'm sorry that you feel so sad.

If you had called I would have been there with both of you. She helped me make sense of all of cancer's horrors and she paid the ultimate price. Down deep I knew it was coming, but there was nothing I could do and I'm still unable to accept that Mimi paid that price and not me.

We didn't know each other then, but we both started out at the same time with the same oncologist. We even had identical symptoms that so many other doctors missed or overlooked. She was a nurse and she played by all the rules and look at the price she paid. I've always been an advocate for myself and here I am with an incurable cancer and I'm actually regaining my health. She helped make all my future happen and now she's gone. It's very painful to face that reality.

When others didn't care, or gave up or said 'Not my job' she did care. In her own quiet way she reached out and calmed the most difficult times, gave me a plan others could have given me but didn't. And now after playing by all the prescribed rules she's gone. Why someone so beautiful and not me? I just don't get it anymore."

With large tears now flooding his eyes, too, Sari said softly, "My turn," and reached over to blot the tears falling across his cheeks.

"As an oncology nurse I've certainly had my share of life's tough transitions and I thought a lot about being there with Mimi in her final hours. In the end I was unable to turn my back. I guess I cared too much. I'd become too emotionally involved. Maybe she meant so much to me because of how much she meant to you. I'm sorry. I'm not making any sense, am I?"

Still looking at her as it was dawning on him how much Sari was becoming his sole cheerleader Penn said, "I'm incredibly grateful to you, but I don't know how to thank you for how you softened this moment for me. After you stopped me from going to see Mimi that last time and told me what I didn't want to hear, I didn't know how I was going to handle her passing. And you put me first. You didn't have to do that. I'm grateful, but I'm just lost for words."

Looking up at him Sari said, "Before you ask, I've decided that I'm not going to Mimi's service. It's just too much for me and I need to get back into my objective nurse mode. Can you understand?"

"I do. I really do and it may be best that you don't go. But I will go to her service. Want me to send flowers from us?" Penn said.

"Can you do it as before, like 'Penn and a Friend'?" Sari asked.

"Sure. If I'm experienced at anything it's sending her those cards, but this time with lots of flowers. Consider it done," he said.

"We need to get back upstairs and get your hydration started. Think anyone will gossip if we walk into the infusion area together looking like a couple of train wrecks?" Sari asked as she began to lighten up.

"Gee. Maybe we should see it as an opportunity. The place always has the same movie playing. Let's give the rest of the audience something it hasn't already seen as a re-run," Penn said while covering her clasped hands with his.

"The café mocha was good," Sari said to lighten-up as she wiped the last tears from her cheeks with her sleeve as they walked across the *Atrium* together and toward the elevators.

After collecting his vital data of weight, temperature, oxygen and blood pressure Penn headed into the infusion area expecting his favorite chair to already be taken. Instead, there was a note taped to the front of his chair that read "Occupied". Since he had not yet been in the infusion area, it could only have come from one person.

As she approached with the IV kit for his hydration and treatment Penn looked into Sari's eyes, as her stoicism was betrayed by the faintest smile.

"Remember, we still need to talk about you getting a port. My head is kind of in another place this morning, so it may have to wait till next time. OK?"

Penn's wordless look back to her said it all.

"Dr. Collins is not in clinic this morning, so I put your ZQT order in for Suzette to sign when I came in. I'll be back soon with your pre-meds and the ZQT should be along soon, too. You look tired, why don't you try to sleep after the pre-meds?" she said with another of her trademark smiles.

Soon she was back with his pre-meds. But this time the Benadryl hit fast and hard and he was quickly fast asleep, so much so that he even slept through the entire ZQT treatment.

As Penn awoke it was to Sari gently pressing his right shoulder. With only a couple other patients left in the infusion area, clearly she could have let him sleep a while longer. But he soon sensed she was on another of her ever present missions.

"Something else I want to share with you before you leave. Can you?" she said quietly.

"Sure. No problem. Here or somewhere else?" Penn said while still trying to get his post-sleep bearings.

"Let's walk over to the 'Garden' and I'll remove the IV line"

The Garden wasn't really a garden, but a large three-sided glass cube off the end of a long corridor where patients could sit in peaceful reflection as they overlooked an outside scene of woodland tranquility from comfortable ochre colored leather chairs. Today it had probably been pre-scouted by Sari, as it was then bathed in soft sunshine and high white clouds, but empty of other patients or their support teams.

"I'm sure I'm breaking a lot of rules by saying this, but both of you have come to mean a lot to me and I need to share something with you. Can you keep this confidential?" Sari began.

"Absolutely, please go ahead."

"I see a lot of people with cancer go past that nurses' station. But, seriously, they're all the same. They just want to get better, to regain their health and go back to their old agendas. They don't really connect cancer's dots. Almost none ever have a real goal or become their own advocate. No heroes, either. They just take orders. But you're different.

Your coloring outside the lines is the reason why you're alive and regaining your health. That's the difference and it's what Mimi saw in you a long time ago. Like when you two first met."

Penn started to say, but Sari raised her hand in a wave of "not now".

"Because she became your mentor she was different in how she reached out to you. She knew that while she wouldn't color outside the lines that you could and her mentoring and encouragement were her gifts to you. Think about that. She saw it in you back when you two first met and Mimi gave you everything she wanted for herself, but knew she couldn't have. It was there in you all the time and Mimi made you see what you had not been able to see in yourself.

I mean, just look in a mirror at you now versus when you walked in here two years ago, then tell me I'm wrong."

With tears now gently falling across her cheeks Sari continued, "Going forward you need to see Mimi in a different way, like the way I'm seeing her in you right here. You're feeling the pain of losing her like I am, too. But Mimi was a very special gift to you."

With more tears and a quiver in her voice she continued, "Do you remember our conversation about your heroes?"

"Yes, sure. Why?" as he nodded yes, but emotionally.

"You were Mimi's hero, you owned all the cards. We became like sisters and we talked a lot. She loved you more than you'll ever know.

As a nurse Mimi knew cancer was a tragedy in three acts. And she could see how hard you were trying to not do Act Three. She so much envied your ability to look at risks and advocate for yourself in fighting your cancer. She loved you so much ... [more emotional sniffles] ... and she never gave up on you.

In losing Mimi you're learning that once you have cancer you never leave the crumple zone of the accident, even after the crash has ended. Like you are now as you're living through your own fate. Mimi's gifts to you were in what she brought out in you. And that's how you are going to get past this crash. Never lose touch with how much she loved you and from that first day you were her hero. To her you were always larger than life.

I so much wish now that I had been willing to break my vow to her that I would not tell you this while there was still time for her. Maybe you could have talked her into becoming an advocate for herself, too. And maybe she would still be alive. It's really painful. I feel like I failed her."

More sniffles as Sari wiped her tears with her sleeve and looked out from the *Garden's* glass walls to the outside sunshine. "Hard as it is for me to be saying this to you, Mimi gave you some things she could only give to you. You're the only one who has walked past that nurses' station who will color outside the lines with the courage to counter-attack an aggressive and incurable cancer. She brought that out in you and they were her gifts to you, even though she wanted them for herself, too

If I sound like I've just made a big fool of myself I'm very sorry, but I just had to share this with you. Please forgive me?"

With tears now filling his eyes, too, while looking into her equally red eyes, "Sari, there's nothing for me to forgive of you. You're the most sincere and beautiful person I know and I ... "

But Sari interrupted him, "Penn, when I stopped you from going over to Mimi that last time it was because I didn't want you to see her so frail and hurt by the cancer. I could see what was likely to happen, as it had for so many others. I knew how much you meant to each other and I just wanted you to remember her as you knew her and because Mimi would have wanted it that way, too.

Now I'm even more convinced it was the right thing to do. Even though Mimi has passed, her spirit and her gifts to you are very much alive in you right now. Please see Mimi for the beautiful gift she was to you and not for the pain of your loss. Don't get in your own way. I know you can do this. Please, for her and for me?"

With uncontrolled tears streaming down his face Penn raised his eyes to hers, "Sari, I can't even begin to describe the pain of losing Mimi. There are no words. There'll be no more gentle kisses to rescue me from being sucked into cancer's crushing black hole, again. And I can't be there for her with an embrace when her next crash happens. Our time together now seems like a candle's brief flicker and yet I am so grateful for every second of Mimi in my life. She truly was a gift. I owe a debt I'll never be able to repay. Never, ever," he said as Sari dabbed his tears with their soggy tissue.

"So you're probably right, but I need some time. I really miss her and yet we were just good friends. But it went much deeper. Maybe she did see something I've been missing. I'm sure you're right about my coloring outside the lines. I've thought for a long time it's helped me make it this far. But, as much as she was my mentor in my cancer journey, you're the only other person who has reached out to me this way.

I know you've got to get back to your other patients, but I owe you a huge thanks for taking this time to be here. Now I've got even more to think about. I guess my coloring outside the lines and advocacy are coming back to haunt me."

"OK [as Sari sniffles and Penn blots her tears again with a tissue]. We'll talk about the port-thing next time. Another mocha?"

With a faint smile, "No, don't want to OD on a good thing. Maybe just a long drive down the coast. See you next time, and thanks."

"I might try to go with you sometime. Oops, shouldn't have said that. Drive carefully, OK?"

"I like your idea. I won't forget."

WIFM - Reality Assessment #11

Replicants weren't supposed to have feelings.
Neither were Blade Runners.

Penn: *It hurts when this happens because it defies everything we want to believe is right in life. It's not supposed to happen this way. But it does happen to very good people. And it's especially painful when it strikes so close.*

Even Sari, with all her objective nurse training, couldn't escape losing someone so close, so innocent as Mimi.

Penn, on the other hand, has a much bigger problem to overcome, especially with no cheerleader at home as one of his support troops. Recall that Mimi was Penn's original mentor, his cheerleader, as he entered cancer's treatment house of horrors in "Cancer: Who Gave Me Cancer?"

And it was Mimi who reached across the divide to guide him through the unknown at each of those initial steps. So Penn is headed for a very rough adjustment to life without Mimi because Mimi was how the training wheels came off for him.

It was Mimi who helped him to take those first tentative steps into his own cancer advocacy. If Penn only had one cheerleader in his life who owned all the chips on the table, it was Mimi.

It's not right and it's not fair, but it is real.

The best we can do is to be prepared by having "My Chronic Cancer" as our strategic goal and "My Cancer Advocacy" as our tactical means. This is how to "Put the How Into Hope" for ourselves and to become stalwart examples to others with cancer. And it's how "to change certainty".

They will not eliminate the pain when we lose someone so close, nor will they change the ruthlessness of cancer.

But they will get us back on the right track as we return to the task of building our next Base Pairs. Penn is ...

<u>BP Score Card</u>:
Ping = 0, Pong = 0, Penn = 3   - *Bad things happen to good people*
- *Cancer doesn't care and it doesn't take prisoners*
- *Keep moving.*

#12 Not Everything That Goes Bump is Cancer

No night. No Day. No Rest.

Ping: Bumps happen, but not every bump will destroy the front-end of your car was Ping's view. In life you just have to be able to tell the difference between a little bump and a terminal bump. Likewise, to Ping cancer's bumps were different, too. Kind of like pot holes. Not every pot hole is terminal to the car, and not every medical bump is cancer. So, net-net, everything can be rationalized!

To Ping cancer's bumps and symptoms are different, like a lot different. To him what's really important is to be aware of the differences between everyday events and cancer's symptoms. That way it's possible to make more progress. After all, life already has too much burdensome overhead and stress. To Ping cancer's bumps were easier to recognize because, "they're always just over the top".

"Though I've had a couple of rounds with bladder cancer I'm doing fine and they can't find any evidence of the cancer, even after six months since the last treatment ended," Ping said to a friend on the phone while at work.

"Right, but that doesn't mean it's not still there," his friend replied.

"I know, but cancer is so different that I'm sure I'll know if it returns again."

"But suppose it doesn't have to return because it's already there now. How would you be able to know in enough time? Even you said the original symptoms seemed like a muscle ache and they turned-out to be bladder cancer. Are you sure it's possible to tell the difference?" his friend asked.

Ping knew this was a line of conversation he was uncomfortable with. And his subconscious knew it was one where Ping had no depth because he was all opinion and no facts.

"Hey, just got another call. Let's catch-up again later. OK?" And, gratefully, the stress of the moment subsided.

Later that afternoon Ping stopped at Dr. Allen's office to get the update from the latest routine CT scan. Dr. Allen had arranged for these updates at six month intervals and today's OV was more a nuisance to Ping because it was too beautiful a day to spend any of it in a doctor's office for something that was an obvious non-starter.

Instead of an exam Dr. Allen just had Ping sit opposite him at his office desk. To Ping the view out the window to a bright sun filled afternoon further reminded him of other places he would rather be. There was absolutely no evidence of the pain or urination frequency he had experienced, either initially or in the subsequent relapses.

Still, Dr. Allen felt he owed Ping the courtesy of the face-to-face meeting. "Let's just not make this an ordeal," Ping thought.

"Good to see you again," Dr. Allen said as they shook hands and sat back into their chairs. "First, how have you been feeling? Any changes since our last meeting?"

"No changes. No pain and my urination frequency is unchanged. Really can't find anything to complain about."

"Are you eating OK? Any changes in your weight or in sleeping?" Dr. Allen asked, probing beyond Ping's first line of defense.

"Appetite is fine, weight is unchanged and I'm sleeping through the night, unlike the last time."

"Good and I'm glad you could make it today. I just received the radiologist's report of the CT scan you had done at the hospital last week. In general the bladder still shows a residual thickness in the same area as all the previous CT scans. The radiologist's thinking is that this thick area is scar tissue from the former cancer. Not a concern, at least at this time.

However, the radiologist did identify a new area on your left ureter about one centimeter above where it enters the bladder. Ureters are the small tubes leading from each kidney to the bladder that pass urine from the kidneys to the bladder. He noted that the area was very small, about 3 mm wide x 5 mm long. This may be nothing, or it could be the emergence of your bladder cancer in a new location, something we call metastasized cancer.

Whatever it is, or isn't, is very early and very small. It may even have been caused by how you were then lying on the CT scanner or due to the orientation of your ureters to other organs. I think that's unlikely, but either way you should be confident that we can move quickly to resolve its true identity," Dr. Allen said.

"Only about 3 millimeters wide x 5 millimeters long! How did he pick this up?" Ping asked in amazement.

"Actually, your scan was read by a new radiologist who recently joined the hospital's staff. The previous radiologist who had read your earlier scans retired about two months ago.

The new radiologist is young, bright and very detailed. He joined the hospital from a large urban cancer hospital and he's really been doing a terrific job in just the past couple of months that he's been on staff. His reports are incredibly detailed and nothing like the one or two lines we would typically get from the radiologist who retired.

Here's the current report that we're discussing now [as Dr. Allen handed Ping the newest report]. The report spans an entire page and addresses the pros and cons of the area. He went back to your most recent CT scan, but could not find any evidence in the same area in your previous scan.

Just for comparison, here's the previous report from the radiologist who recently retired. Just three lines and no comparison to your previous CT scan. Quite a difference," Dr. Allen concluded as he was then moving-on.

"I agree with the report and believe we should move quickly to determine the true nature of the finding. You'll see at the bottom of the report the new radiologist suggested a PET-CT scan for two good reasons. First, it would be a different type of scan of the same area; and second, it would specifically determine if any cancer exists in your bladder and in the ureter.

If you're OK with this approach, and I believe it's the right next step, we can schedule you for the PET-CT scan next week? It will take about an hour."

"The questions never stop do they?" Ping said reflectively, "Let's go ahead and schedule the scan. Give me a call and let me know the date and time, preferably in the early AM."

"Good," Dr. Allen said as they both stood-up and shook hands in departure. Dr. Allen could see that Ping was still puzzled by the discussion of the new area and the upcoming PET-CT scan.

Pong: In Pong's dysfunctional cancer awareness his conscious focus was on what was happening then, not on if-then-else.

In his mindset nearly everything that could not be readily explained as being non-cancerous was therefore guilty of having a cancer association before it could be deemed innocent. When looked at through such a lens everything becomes tarred by the same brush, but still not part of the bigger picture.

Pong was approaching his six month post-treatment review for which Dr. Black had scheduled a follow-up PET-CT scan. For the scan Pong arrived early hoping to get a jump on others who might be running a bit late. In that respect he was right. So the radiology team moved him ahead of those who had been scheduled ahead of Pong, but had not yet arrived. To Pong it seemed like his time on the scanner table was less than the previous scan and he was soon on to other important things on his to-do list.

Two days later he was again face-to-face with Dr. Black and the PET-CT scan report of Dr. Bernstein.

Dr. Black began, "Well, Pong, Dr. Bernstein's report is quite interesting to say the least."

"What does that mean?" Pong asked somewhat puzzled.

"It means that according to the PET-CT scan you did two days ago there's both bad news and good news. Let me advise you of the bad news first. The bad news, such as it is in Dr. Bernstein's report, is that you still appear to have melanoma in the tissue surrounding the original patches on your back and the metastasized melanoma in those two spots on your lungs for which you did the Interleukin and radiation treatments. As bad news goes in melanoma, that's not as bad as it could be.

Then, the good news is that the patches on your back are unchanged from the previous PET-CT scan and the same can be said for the two spots on your lungs. Dr. Bernstein indicated that none of those areas appear to have undergone any change in growth or in shrinkage.

The other good news is that Dr. Bernstein can find no evidence in the PET-CT scan of your melanoma having metastasized to any other area, such as your lymph nodes. And that's really good news because melanoma has a nasty habit of doing just that. Blink and it's sprouted somewhere else."

"I'm confused. Do I still have melanoma or is it gone? I've had some other symptoms and I thought they were melanoma, too?" Pong asked.

"Pong, as elusive as this might be, please don't mistake my enthusiasm for the realities of dealing with melanoma as a patient. The melanoma is still there and in the same locations, but it has not increased in size in those locations and it is surprising us by not showing up elsewhere," Dr. Black said.

"Ok then, I have some other symptoms, let's call them 'bumps' that I'd like to check-out with you. The first is a spot on my right forearm. It's brown and I'm concerned it could be more of the same original melanoma?"

Inspecting the spot on Pong's right forearm Dr. Black responded, "This spot is actually just the kind of brown spots we accrue as we age. This spot is somewhat larger than most others on your skin, but its shape is quite regular, it has no height, its color is all consistent. In my opinion it is just a brown spot that is darker than others and not at all unusual for someone like you with a fair complexion."

"So, it's not cancerous and not a concern?"

"Not at all. Anything else?"

"Yes. I was out for a walk a few days ago and thought I had become more winded than was normal for me."

"Pong, if you're thinking those two spots on your lungs are indicative of an advancing malignancy that will quickly impair your breathing ability in routine exercise please do not do so. First, both spots are incredibly small and most likely have no ability to be such an impairment. Second, you'll do yourself a lot more good than harm by continuing to exercise.

Please understand that there are bumps and there are cancerous bumps. You should continue to bring your concerns to me just as we are discussing them right now, but do not try to read too much into any one bump or event. It's very safe to say that 99.9% of all bumps in life are not cancer. But to say that to cancer patients does not ring the same as saying it to people who do not have cancer."

"So, you're saying..." as Pong interrupted Dr. Black.

"Right. I'm saying that you should always feel free to ask me about any particular symptom. No exceptions. And you should never feel any hesitation. But don't be surprised that nearly all of them are unlikely to have any affiliation to your cancer. Does that help?"

"Sure does. Makes a huge difference. When should we meet again?"

"Let's make sure this stays under our microscope. Let's meet again in thirty days. We'll have the benefit of having allowed the IL-2 and the radiation to have fully impacted all the sites and we can make a more rational plan at that time," Dr. Black concluded.

"Fine with me. I'm glad you have a plan," Pong said in relief.

Penn: No matter how he had tried to prepare himself or how much Sari had rationalized life's realities, losing Mimi to cancer

205

was a huge loss and he was making little progress getting out of his slump from losing her.

Yet, ironic as it may seem, the cyclic re-occurrence of his NHL symptoms made it possible for Penn to prevail over the experiences of depression and other distractions that would have been major hurdles to others. Cancer has its own way of relentlessly securing the top spot on our to-do lists.

Even after his wife had served notice of her decision to move to her sister's in Charleston, to his surprise he had kind-of recovered from her leaving in part because his NHL symptoms became a perpetual reminder of cancer's priority. But losing Mimi was a different matter entirely. Losing Mimi became the tipping-point in his life because Mimi had become his center of gravity.

Penn knew that Mimi had succumbed for the same reasons his other cancer friends had succumbed to cancer, but "why not me?" still did not compute. And this had become a 24x7 haunting. Even against Sari's emotional appeals, he became unable to escape her loss. It pursued him everywhere.

He had tried evenings alone with some solitary music. That created more problems than it solved. He tried long drives in the Porsche up into the mountains and along the coast, but returning home he was still faced with the same impasse. Even dinners with lots of wine didn't work either. But it did shorten the evenings!

Fortunately, if that's possible to say, his ZQT treatments were a repeatable change of pace and back into familiar territory. Like the place had become his second home.

Arriving for his next ZQT treatment at 8 AM he was expecting to be met by Sari, but he soon learned that hearing her now familiar soft accent would be broken, at least for today's treatment. Sari had left a note that she had been abruptly scheduled into a training class for a new infusion pump and was unlikely to return before he finished his treatment. She had arranged for Elaine to be his nurse today. Penn read the note for Sari's unspoken agenda because he already knew that Elaine had also been Mimi's nurse when Sari was unavailable.

"With her there's always a script. Always. Maybe that's why ... No Penn, don't go there," he began to think to himself as he finished reading Sari's note with a wry smile.

After a few moments, just before his 8:30 AM appointment, Penn heard Elaine call his name. Elaine did not have Sari's soft Mediterranean accent. In fact, Elaine was what Sari was not.

Elaine was efficient and pleasant, but there was no chance Elaine would ever be competition for Sari. It had occurred to Penn that Sari was keenly aware of this, especially when it came to the behind the scenes jockeying that took place between the nurses in this hospital. After as many treatments as he had had at so many hospitals he had become keenly aware of how each hospital's operations took-on their own unique, but recognizable personae.

Whether this hospital operated on the concept of virtual teams or not was beside the point. The real point was, as is universally true, a rule having been ordained by management is not the same as it being followed or enforced to get the job done by the troops in the trenches.

Even thinking back to that first day, standing at the nurses' station for the first time, something had clicked with Sari. After all, she was already very busy and could have easily ignored the opportunity to take on responsibility for one more very challenged cancer patient. Her eyes had given away that truth.

So Elaine became her proxy. Elaine was Sari's non-threat du-jour nurse – a trustable understudy – to ensure no interlopers jumped her claim, and that her patient did not have the chance to wander a-field while she was unavailable.

As Elaine completed the IV hook-up to his hydration, Penn watched with the perspective of a surveyor rechecking his most recent courses and bearings. Elaine always got the job done and she would certainly report back to Sari all her observations from the field on this patient and that patient in addition to all the formal reporting required by the hospital to meet its fiduciary responsibilities.

But what really mattered was the informal report that Sari would extract from Elaine. Penn had resolved that in her report there would be nothing of a "remarkable" nature. He knew well enough to let sleeping puppies nap.

After his hydration had been started, but before his pre-meds arrived Suzette, Dr. Collins' PA, stopped at his infusion chair to inquire if there had been any changes in his appetite, weight, sleep or other routine functions and to let him know that Dr. Collins would likely stop by, too.

To Penn this was an unforeseen opportunity because he had been experiencing some new symptoms and the timing was right to open a discussion of what they could mean. Were they new signs of maturation occurring in his NHL cancer, or the emergence of a collateral cancer, or of a metastasizing of the cancer out of his lymphatic system and into his organs?   To Penn almost any symptom was always tagged as suspect and part of the larger picture before it could be deemed innocent.

As had become his custom, Penn headed over to the small kitchen area to make a cup of coffee. The coffee's caffeine had become essential to head-off the onset of the sleepiness of the Benadryl that was certain to arrive with his pre-meds.

While a bit heads-down and oblivious to others in the area Dr. Collins approached from behind him, "I haven't had my caffeine today either, can you make two of those?"

Looking-up with a smile Penn responded, "This one is yours, just add the cream."

"Didn't mean to ..." Dr. Collins said.

"Not at all. Welcome to my second home."

"You like it here don't you?" Dr. Collins asked.

"Yes, I truly do. You and your team have saved my life. I've made so many new friends that it does feel like a second home."

"If your coffee is ready let's head over to the exam room," Dr. Collins said.

"How have you been feeling? Any new side effects from the ZQT treatments? Your weight seems to be steady, how is your appetite and how are you sleeping?" Dr. Collins asked, as if echoing Suzette's questions.

Penn already knew from past conversations that Dr. Collins often asked several questions at a time and then waited for the patient to respond. "No problems with the ZQT treatments. Whatever issues existed at the outset seem to have been resolved and I have no complaints. My weight seems to be stable and my appetite is fine. I can eat anything, although preferably with red wine," Penn said with a smile.

"Please don't quote me, but I approve of the red wine. How about your sleep? Anything to report, like waking with night sweats?" Dr. Collins asked while examining the lymph nodes in Penn's neck.

"Sleep has become a problem. It's not unusual to wake at 3AM and not be able to get back to sleep until 4 AM, but no night sweats," Penn replied.

"That's good news. I can't explain why you wake-up in the middle of the night, unless if it were due to a symptom like night sweats, which you're not having. Let's watch the sleeping pattern and see if something else develops. I think there is no linkage to your cancer, but let's put it on our to-do list to discuss again in the future. Anything else to report?"

"Yes. Well, sort-of.

The itching is continuing, but in a different pattern on my lower legs. I've developed a red rash on my chest and I have what seems like a perpetual sore throat. Do any of these sound like symptoms you've seen in the past for this cancer or a related cancer?" Penn replied.

"Let's take them one at a time, OK?" Examining Penn's chest just below his throat, then looking into his throat Dr. Collins said, "Let's look at those itchy areas [Penn was able to identify two itchy red spots on his lower legs].

"Are you concerned about these symptoms because you think they may be new cancer symptoms, because you're not sure, or is it due to something else?" Dr. Collins asked.

"Maybe it's because by now I don't know how to not be my own advocate, but I've learned out of my past failure to pay attention and to bring them to your attention."

"OK. I understand and I want you to know that you are doing the right thing to bring these symptoms to my attention. Don't ever let anyone persuade you to do otherwise."

I would break the symptoms into two categories, those that are indicators of your continuing malignancy and those that are indicative of non-cancer conditions. Let's start with the non-cancerous symptoms first.

The red rash and the sore throat are not cancer symptoms. They're almost certainly due to something you've eaten or drank to which you have a mild allergy. Likely not something that would cause a throat closure, but more likely something that you are not yet aware of as being allergic. One of the possibilities is the dexamethasone we give you as a pre-med to reduce the inflammatory effects of the ZQT. Let's substitute two 200 mg ibuprophen for the dexamethasone and see if the red rash and the sore throat resolve by your next ZQT treatment. OK?" Dr. Collins said.

Penn was still in a daze as Dr. Collins said with a smile, "Penn that was a question."

"Oh, yes. I see your point. Let's do that. I won't miss the dexamethasone at all. Maybe my sleep will improve, too."

"Good. You may be right about the sleep. Steroids like dexamethasone are notorious for disrupting sleep patterns, but you already know that from your use of prednisone early-on in your experience with this cancer. I'll remove the dexamethasone from your pre-meds for the next two treatments.

But the itchy red spots on your legs, those are continuing symptoms of your cancer. The fact that those spots are continuing is a reliable indicator of the cancer's persistence. But the declining frequency and the declining severity are both reliable indicators that the ZQT is gaining control over the cancer and not vice-a-versa, such as when you first arrived here.

You should be proud of your accomplishments. You've made real progress and I am increasingly of the opinion that one day you will be able to transition to some form of a maintenance plan.

That does not mean you will ever be cured of this cancer, but it may be possible for the ZQT to control the cancer so you can go back to leading a more normal life," Dr. Collins concluded.

"Thanks for the praise, but it really belongs to this team at this hospital and especially to you and to Sari. It's not lost on me," Penn said in response to Dr. Collins.

"OK, I'll accept your expression of appreciation and I'll pass it on to Sari. But you need to see that without your advocacy none of this progress would have happened. Even your persistence to identify these symptoms, be they cancerous or non-cancerous, has been critical to what has been achieved and you should be proud of your contribution. After all, we need that in our patients for us to create survivors. It's much rarer than you might think.

You're doing fine. Let's see - Sari's not here today - so I need to get you back to Elaine for your pre-meds and your ZQT treatment," Dr. Collins said to close their OV.

WIFM - Reality Assessment #12

Right, no rest. Its vigilance that builds strength.

Ping: *He went into the OV with Dr. Allen with no enthusiasm for getting a real status update. Whether there were new bladder cancer symptoms or not, his mind was elsewhere. It should have been on the update. After all, that was the purpose of the OV.*

The new radiologist produced a more detailed report that indicated the likely presence of metastasized bladder cancer on one of his ureters. But Ping's persistent detachment from the chronic nature of his cancer has walled him off from the implied risks. His lack of education and lack of advocacy have confined him to being unprepared.

He is still unable to discern or understand a minor non-malignant symptom from a malignant symptom. This leaves him unable to maintain a meaningful discussion with his doctor and unable to comprehend the gravitational differences of the previous radiologist vs. the newer radiologist's greater competence. This movie is painful to watch.

Pong: *The most recent PET-CT scan more clearly showed the evolving risks of metastasized melanoma on his lungs. While the two spots are small, their risks are huge.*

Pong is slowly engaging in his on-going symptoms management, e.g. the brown spot on his arm and his being winded during exercise. But the spots detected by the PET-CT scan are being left to a future date to see if the Il-2 and radiation treatments will eventually resolve them. Ouch!!!.

Sure, the non-malignant symptoms do not need further attention, but an aggressive, metastasized cancer like melanoma should not be left to a casual thirty day holiday.

Penn: *By maintaining a log of his symptoms – in his health journal - Penn arrived at the OV with Dr. Collins prioritized and prepared. It signaled to Dr. Collins that Penn was serious and that their time together would be well utilized. By this time in their relationship Dr. Collins knew what to expect of Penn so as to eliminate wasting time.*

Penn's informed advocacy is a key mindset factor to talented professionals, like Dr. Collins, who are always in demand.

With Penn operating as his own educated advocate they were able to cleave the symptoms Penn had logged into malignant and non-malignant. Together they were able to have a closer, more meaningful relationship and to focus on the chronic nature of Penn's NHL sub-type cancer.

Clearly we are seeing Penn increasingly able to function as the 3rd leg of the three legged stool, i.e. the cancer patient, with his resources and technology. *This makes him unlikely to fall down by surprise.*

BP Score Card:
Ping = 0, Pong = 1, Penn = 2 – On-going awareness of all symptoms is key in cancer.
– Develop the honesty to accept the realities of change when living with cancer.

#13 Remission is Not Cancer Free & Maintaining Sustainability

The journey is the reward.

Ping: Silver bullets are great if they really do destroy our adversaries, but often they are just escapes of fantasy. While they allow us to fantasize about the possibilities of eradicating our implacable foes, they carry high costs in the time and distractions they extract.

Having already been through multiple remission-relapse cycles for his bladder cancer, Dr. Allen's news of a new cancer area on his left ureter should be cause for alarm of a likely metastasized condition. Instead, because he could not actually feel the effects of the new area, the gravity of the news made little impact on Ping. "So, maybe its just a shadow?" as he began his rationalization process.

After leaving Dr. Allen's office Ping re-thought the conversation about the radiologist's report. Stopping at the *Starbucks* across the park from *Café Soleil* it was still on his mind, especially the part about how it might have been due to how he was then laying on the scanner's bed during the scan.

"Gee, that technology is really great, maybe too great. If it can see something as small as only about 3 mm x 5 mm, but it can't tell the difference between a shadow and a tumor [as he ignored Dr. Allen's doubt about the shadow], maybe it can't be all that great.

So, if it's small and because of how I was lying at the time, I guess I'm still in remission. Just doesn't make sense that it's anything else. I don't have any pains or any other symptoms. Maybe someone else would get all worked-up over what Dr. Allen said. I just don't see any reason to chase this thing any further.

If he really wants me to do the PET-CT scan, OK. But sure seems like a waste of time."

Ping just did what some of us do with the news about cancer's natural maturation process, i.e. metastasized tumors. We rationalize it into a non-real reality. In cancer situations this can be a very high risk delusion.

Recall that Ping cycles along a predictable pathway of denial-detachment-complacency-to-depression. Ping used the coffee break moment to do his own misguided regression analysis into now familiar territory. Having never put forth the effort to develop either his goal of cancer as a chronic condition nor his own advocacy to achieve that goal, why should we expect anything more of him?

This leaves Ping squarely in the cross-hairs of being unprepared for his next relapse, yet still not pro-actively in control of his future. While his non-cancer-free remission is likely to end soon, even armed with the new news from Dr. Allen, Ping is headed in the wrong direction. Sound familiar?

Pong: While Ping's ability to rationalize away the maturation of the bladder cancer is regrettable, it is nonetheless predictable of him and cancer patients like Ping.

But Pong's most recent conversation with Dr. Black continued to run as a background task in his engineer's mind. "If the melanoma is in decline, why do I still have the spots on both lungs and in the tissue on my back? If the melanoma is shrinking, after this much time why is it still detectable by the PET-CT scan?"

To Pong these questions were like engineering problems he had seen many times; problems that were said to have been solved, but they still produced reoccurring error conditions no one could explain. Like, because no one connected the dots. Hello!

He was beginning to feel that Dr. Black's bad news was really bad and there was more bad than good in the good news.

And to his credit he knew he had already been here before, like when he had inadvertently skied into that couloirs. Too quickly he had passed any hope of a safe exit. He was alone and facing some really bad options – just like now.

Continuing his thinking about the OV with Dr. Black, he decided that the moment was "Now" and a time-out was needed to organize his thoughts. So he placed his cell phone clearly in sight on his desk next to a "Back soon" yellow sticky note and walked from his office over to a quiet area of the plant where he could be alone and just not available for a while.

Going over the conversation with Dr. Black he thought, "Overall the news was neither as good nor as bad as it could have been. But, realistically, it just had the feel that it might be my last wake-up call.

If there was good news in the OV with Dr. Black it had to be in knowing those other symptoms were not related to the melanoma. So that news really does feels good. Then, if all the news about the melanoma spots really was bad news at least now there's a way to separate the two, like ... not everything that goes bump is cancer.

Still, the melanoma has spread and it's persistent, can't deny those facts. We know where it is today and we know it will spread more in the future and then it will spread some more till ... Christ, I've got to get control of this, like now, before it totally owns my future.

This really is like that couloirs all over again. I need to focus on getting the melanoma under control ASAP. Like now!

Right, but how and where? I've been at this so long and I feel like even after this much time and all the treatments in some ways I'm still a novice. This shouldn't be. I've got to do more before it's too late. Don't want to compromise the relationship with Dr. Black, but ...

Wait a minute. Dammit! The answer has been in front of me all along. Penn has been at this cancer-thing a lot longer than either me or Ping. He's actually been through a lot more than either of us and each time we've had lunch we look at him in amazement. I need a heart-to-heart conversation with Penn.

The solution, or the next step to a solution, has to have been in my face all the time. And it's why I've always wanted to arrive early for our lunches, so Penn and I could spend a few minutes together before Ping gets there.

I'm going back to the office and I'm going to call Penn. We need to meet. I'm sure he already has answers to questions I still don't even know how to ask. We could meet at *Un Bel Di* and maybe I can get him to go for a drive to the coast in his Porsche. Damn, this has been there all along. Should have done this a long time ago."

Penn: Just as Ping was doing his misguided regression analysis of Dr. Allen's discussion of the spot on his ureter, and as Pong was reaching his Eureka moment over his recent PET-CT scan, Penn was awaiting the next OV with Dr. Collins and the start of his next treatment ZQT cycle.

Sari met him at the reception desk, walked him past the nurses' station and into the infusion area, collected his vital signs and started his hydration. But as she started the pump for the hydration she said, with a hint or defense, "I've got to attend a review class in another area of the hospital. It will probably take till mid-afternoon, so I can't be back before you finish your ZQT treatment.

I've already asked Elaine to take over for me. She'll take care of your pre-meds and get you to see Dr. Collins and the ZQT treatment. You'll do fine. See you next time. OK?" she said, but more as a statement than as a question.

Penn knew that statements ending as questions and questions ending as statements are inherently the same things: preludes to hidden agendas. While he had confidence in Sari, Elaine too, he had become accustomed to his routine and the absence of the perpetual Hell that had preceded his arrival as a patient of Dr. Collins and Sari. If the hospital's management had just asked him, though not at all likely, he would have re-scheduled Sari's class to another day.

Penn had learned about busy doctors in general, and Dr. Collins in particular, that really good doctors are always in demand and very busy. If his OV with Dr. Collins had been scheduled for later than 10 AM he knew he could wait a long time for the OV to start because Dr. Collins' time would already be running behind with other patients elsewhere in the hospital.

While he had often heard patients grouse about their long waits to see their doctors, he knew the waiting time to see really good doctors, like Dr. Collins and others at this cancer hospital, was a non-issue. Don't take it personal. Just plan ahead with a book or work on a computer and be appreciative of their availability regardless of the time spent waiting.

After a lengthy delay Penn could detect Dr. Collins voice in the hallway with another doctor, followed by Dr. Collins arrival in the exam room with, "Hi, sorry I'm so late."

"Not a problem. I brought some things to read so I was able to get some work done until you arrived."

"OK, just sit on the exam table so I can check your lymph nodes and listen to your lungs," as Dr. Collins proceeded with a routine exam.

"On my way here I picked-up your labs from today's blood draw. I've also reviewed the results of the flow cytometry we ran on your last blood draw from the previous ZQT treatment. Today's blood results look just like all your other recent results so that's good news. It means your condition has stopped changing, which can happen with your NHL sub-type, such as if the cancer had spread to your organs or if the disease was undergoing maturation because it was not under control.

As far as the flow cytometry results are concerned we're seeing very consistent results from one to another, and we've run the flow cytometry many times on your blood. If I were to put all this into a summary for you it would argue that your NHL sub-type cancer is now under control. Under the current ZQT treatment regimen it is not able to advance, but we are not able to declare you cancer-free either.

Based on your most recent PET-CT scan it is undetectable and we believe we are able to prevent it from maturing past your immune system. We are now able to kill all the emergent malignant cells the ZQT can identify at each treatment," Dr. Collins concluded.

Penn saw the opportunity and asked, "You've said I am not cancer-free, but you've also gone to a substantial effort to assess the state of my cancer. Is there more?"

"Yes, there is more and I'm glad you are able to ask that question. I am of the opinion that you are now able to transition to a maintenance plan with the ZQT just as you are here for today, but on a new schedule of once every two weeks. Starting today.

I've discussed this plan with my colleagues and we all concur in that conclusion. But, first, I want to ask you if you are OK with our plan? Before you answer you should know that we will be watching you just as we are now and you will reporting back to me at the start of each ZQT cycle, just as we are doing today.

If your results appear to be trending negative for any reason we will not hesitate to immediately return to the present ZQT treatment regimen so that you do not regress further. What do you think of our analysis and our plan?"

"I guess it's obvious I'm overcome by emotion just now, so please forgive me but I ... [recovering, Penn then said] When I became a patient of you not that long ago I had a deadly cancer that had left me with no chips. In that time you, this team and the ZQT have actually given me back my health and my life. And just now you've described how you and your colleagues have actually been monitoring my progress in such detail that you have confidence I am strong enough to transition to a ZQT-based maintenance plan, like I have nothing more than a treatable chronic condition.

[Again, overcome by emotion] This is just incredible. Obviously I'm going to say 'Yes', but I need to pinch myself to believe all this is really happening. I just never never thought it possible this moment would ever happen. Never in my wildest dreams."

"Penn your NHL sub-type is very rare and aggressive. That combination in cancer more often than not leads to high mortality rates. Combine them with the cancer also being incurable and those mortality rates usually increase exponentially. So to prevail over your cancer, as you have so far, requires that the patient engage as his or her own advocate.

Thus, what one of your earlier oncologists told you about you likely succumbing to the cancer within the initial two to three years from the onset of symptoms is regrettable, but statistically accurate. You probably did not like his candor at the time, but you can now look back on his comment in awe of its accuracy vs. what you've achieved.

As you evolved your advocacy to reach a cancer-centric hospital like ours with this team, you actually placed yourself in the care of a team with deep experience with your NHL cancer sub-type. That is what made it possible for us to lock-into your cancer with the ZQT treatment and to configure the ZQT treatment to attack your cancer. Your advocacy and our team with the ZQT are what have made your new maintenance plan possible.

You may not know this, but you are my longest surviving patient with this NHL sub-type. In fact, look at it this way: while we have an exceptional team of medical professionals at this cancer hospital with absolutely the most advanced resources and medical technology that includes very advanced medicines, all of that would have meant nothing to you, nor to me, if you had not become your own advocate and made your way here to be my patient.

In other words, Penn, without you as your own advocate striving to become a patient here and without you striving every day to prevail over your cancer you would have died about two years ago and none of our team, none of our resources and none of our medicines would have been of any value to you. I would not be having this conversation with you.

So thank you for your praise and I am truly honored to be here with you at this moment. But it's you and your advocacy that are what made this moment happen. I truly wish there were more patients like you. You should be extremely proud of what you've accomplished."

"Thank you for that praise, but I am still in shock and almost can't believe its true," Penn replied, but in awe of Dr. Collins candor.

"So, you now have a new schedule and some free time to think about. Let's get you back to Elaine. I guess Sari is away at a training class, and Elaine will get you started on your ZQT treatment," Dr. Collins said to begin moving past Penn's emotion of the moment.

WIFM - Reality Assessment #13

In cancer it's all in how we manage the journey
that determines whether we change certainty.

Ping: *People like Ping just defy reason. Given a simple fact they will frustrate us with their propensity to rationalize that 2+2≠5.*

Even if he does not like the news in the radiologist's report – none of us would - that his bladder cancer has metastasized to one of his ureters, he is setting himself for a crash when the upcoming PET-CT scan refutes his misguided conclusion about the origin of the new area. Furthermore, Ping has consistently second guessed the medical profession's advancing technology with a solid no-wins track record.

It's incredible that likeable people, like Ping, really are able to convince themselves they are more informed than their doctors with advanced technology.

We should also observe that Dr. Allen first ordered a CT scan. He did not order a PET-CT scan. At 3 mm x 5 mm the PET-CT scan would have likely identified the new area as a metastasized tumor, thus settling its status and being able to a move to a treatment plan sooner. Another baseline opportunity missed. So Ping has to endure the PET-CT scan as a second scan with the additional radiation.

Here we go, again, into another relapse. One has to ask, how much can someone like Ping absorb before they - we - can absorb no more and the cancer gains the advantage, which it is always trying to do? Ping needs to be on the offense and he's barely playing defense.

Pong: *In William Faulkner's "The Bear", Ike must give-up his safety net of distractions for Ben, the bear, to allow the two of them to meet.*

Like Ike, and after so much futile effort, Pong has resolved to come face-to-face with what has been stalking him for so long. But to do so he must abandon his safety net by willfully placing his electronic gadgets, i.e. his distractions, out of his reach and confronting his own fears so he can face his own cancer adversary one-on-one. This can be scary turf.

By doing so Pong found a resource that had been accessible to him for much longer than he would like to admit - Penn, his friend. Penn had already made a lot of progress against a very difficult cancer. But until this moment he had not tapped into Penn's experience.

Put in very bottom-line terms, if Pong is able to quickly and effectively leverage Penn's chronic cancer advocacy experience to his advantage he may still have a chance for his survival.

If he does not, against an adversary like metastasized melanoma, his chances of survival will rapidly decline - as cancer gains the advantage. ***Again its offense, offense, offense.***

Penn: *It's true, remission is not the same as cancer-free.*

Penn attained his long sought strategic goal of reaching a state of "My Chronic Cancer" because he continuously developed his own "My Cancer Advocacy". Along the way he had as many, if not more, serious failures of treatments, failed doctor relationships and OJCT [On the Job Cancer Training] events as Ping and Pong combined.

Penn prevailed because he learned how to become the third leg of the three-legged stool - patient, resources and technology - by setting his chronic cancer goal and developing his own cancer advocacy. As he made progress against a rare, aggressive and incurable cancer he also achieved something else. He developed and accumulated a new confidence in himself that he could mount an effective offensive campaign and see it through to success. That was the source of his emotion in the OV with Dr. Collins.

And let's give credit to Penn's primary team, too. Comprehensive cancer hospitals and medical professionals like Dr. Collins and Sari and technologies like ZQT do exist and more are becoming available all the time. But we cannot expect them to find us. We must set our goals and become our own advocates to find and work with them.

That is, in cancer we must always be on the offense and always be our own advocates.

BP Score Card:
Ping = 0, Pong = 1, Penn = 3 - Remission is not a proxy for cancer
free.
- Fantasy is always costly and delusional in cancer.
- The only impossibility is the one we will not do.

#14 To All Things There is a Season

Make a dent in cancer's universe.

Penn: This Saturday AM Penn delayed getting-up and just lay in bed till about 9, staring up at the ceiling while getting nowhere with ideas of how to fill his new day. Still feeling aimless he took a shower and dressed, but could find nothing of interest for breakfast.

Re-thinking the day, and the absence of any real commitments to accomplish anything, while shaving he decided that a café mocha, a chocolate croissant and the *"Times"* on the terrace at *Un Bel Di* were the best ways to start the day. "Yes! Just do it," he directed to his silent opposite staring back at him from inside the mirror.

On the short drive to *Un Bel Di* he turned on the radio and realized the last time he had driven the Porsche he left the radio tuned to a satellite music station. The song just then being played was Peter, Paul and Mary's *"If I had a Hammer"*. It was at that moment the gravity of the conversation with Dr. Collins hit home.

Along with Dr. Collins and Sari and Dr. Collins' ZQT magic potion he had actually dented cancer's universe. It was at that moment he knew as his own cancer advocate he had actually become the third leg of the proverbial three legged stool and the conversation with Dr. Collins about the transition to the ZQT maintenance plan was the reason why this Saturday AM was so different. "Damn right tune! Penn, you've earned this mocha," he declared to the topless Porsche.

The Saturday AM terrace at *Un Bel Di* is almost always in fog and usually only sparsely peopled by those bipeds truly lacking in near term agendas. After all, who else would want to sit outside in a fog?

Except for an occasional skateboarder or a mom with a three wheeled carriage, it's usually deserted. Arriving at 10 he realized his first non-decision decision of the day was perfect.

He soon had the Porsche parked, gotten his café mocha with a double espresso, a chocolate croissant and the *Times*.

"Now, if I just had that WFT Sari has been pestering me about I'd have a soul mate to commiserate with," he pondered as he opted for a small white marble topped bistro table with two chairs tucked under one of the building's red awnings with a propane heater. Truthfully, the fog and the heat felt great.

"I was about to order something when I saw you out here on the terrace and alone and I wasn't sure if I should come over or say anything. I don't know if you're expecting company, or have other plans. But I, I mean I …"

Looking up to the voice he already knew so well, Penn was speechless as he looked into the beautiful azure eyes of the only person who could have spoken those words in that soft accent. Somehow, out of the fog, Sari had just filled the day with everything that was not yet there. As she spoke Penn knew this was a true gift.

"I have no impending guests, no scheduled appointments. Don't even have that wire fox terrier, at least not yet. But I am grateful to have beautiful company. You're welcome to join me, but only if I can buy you a café mocha. Please say, 'Yes'," he said with a warm smile.

"I guess I'm the tourist now. Maybe I shouldn't …" she said, as if caught in her own solo moment of self-doubt.

"Please Sari [gesturing to the empty chair]. I can't tell you how happy I am to see you [rising and giving her a one armed hug]. Please sit here [again, gesturing to the open chair]. I'll get your mocha and be right back," leaving her no chance to reconsider.

Returning with the café mocha and the muffin du-jour Penn began, "What a treat..." but Sari interrupted.

"Didn't sleep much last night and with it being Saturday I was just kind of wandering and you had said such nice things about this place that I just thought I'd ... but I didn't mean to interrupt ..."

"Sari, your showing-up like this is a dream come true. Please forget the second thoughts, the apologies and any excuse to find something else to do. Please cancel everything you had on today's to-do list. I've just declared that today is just for us."

"I still feel kind of guilty, I ..."

"Sari [Penn leans forward and crosses the line with a gentle kiss on Sari's cheek] you're the most beautiful person in the world and this is our day. Isn't a mocha in the fog at *Un Bel Di* wonderful?"

Sari's look said it all. She now knew why she had wandered to *Un Bel Di*. "I probably don't have to tell you what's been on my mind, do I?" she said in soft reflection.

"Truly, you don't. I know why you didn't sleep last night. It's been on mine, too. I think we're both better at 'Hello' than 'Goodbye'. You were right. Mimi was an irreplaceable friend. But with you here I'm able to set it aside. I'm so happy you're here. Even in this fog, you've just brightened the day. This day is truly ours," Penn said softly while looking into her eyes.

"So you're OK with me ...?

"I couldn't be happier. How's the mocha and muffin?"

"Please don't tell my other patients, but their great. I didn't sleep much last night. Did I already say that? And you had talked about how much you like this place. Oh, I said that too, didn't I? I just thought I'd give it a try. That's when I saw you out here on the terrace and, well, I guess you know the rest. What's the muffin?"

"Morning Glory. Over the top healthy and goes great with a mocha. Might even pass Charlie's scrutiny."

With a smile Sari changed the subject. "I heard the good news from Dr. Collins. You must be pleased?" she said from under her wide brim straw hat, while looking at him from behind the rim of the warm café mocha that she cradled with both hands,

"I sure wish you could have been there,"

"Well, it really was about what you and Dr. Collins have accomplished since you arrived," she said with a hint of defense.

"OK, there was that to the moment with Dr. Collins, but you were indispensable to the journey. I'll never stop being grateful to you.

When I first walked in to our hospital I was experienced at gaining access to cancer treatments, but still naïve. In a space of about two years I had had so many treatments and they were all failures, both for the treatments as well as the relationships.

Along the way I'd learned to become my own advocate. But I never stopped to realize there's a limit to how much chemo our bodies can take. It truly had become a St. Vitas Dance.

To stay alive I'd become a steroid and chemo junkie. When I arrived as a patient of Dr. Collins and you that first day, as the

229

previous clinical trial was failing so badly, I was hoping for success but also prepared to move on to the next treatment when the ZQT failed, as I expected it would. For a lot of reasons I'm glad it succeeded.

It's actually taken me a long time to see that it really is possible for cancer patients to advocate for themselves and to find the right teams and the right treatments to prevail over their cancers. But it does take commitment and the ability to believe in ourselves.

So, yes, I am very pleased Dr. Collins has enough confidence that I can transition to a maintenance plan, even if it means being on ZQT every two weeks indefinitely. But, in truth, it wasn't me. It was you and Dr. Collins who pulled off this incredible accomplishment. Wasn't possible without you."

"Thanks, you're very kind," Sari said with new depth to her eyes and a blush she was unable to hide, still cradling the mocha.

Looking at her through the ever present softness in her voice, Penn was then in awe of the transformation then taking place between them. He was seeing Sari in a different way, like she was the most beautiful person in the world and someone he did not want to ever leave.

With Acker Bilk's soft clarinet solo *"Feelings"* gently drifting over *Un Bel Di's* now sun dappled terrace, Penn knew in his heart this moment had been a long time coming. While he sometimes saw other nurses for his ZQT treatments, from that first day at the nurses' station it had always been different with Sari.

She nearly always greeted him at the reception desk. She collected his vital signs at the start of each treatment and she quietly ran interference when the hospital's administrivia machine broke down – usually at the worst possible of times. She put the

IV in his arm and said "Sorry" each time. Then she gently put the bandage on the IV wound at the end of each ZQT treatment. She bird-dogged him about the "port-thing" and she always checked his idiot mittens and sun block! And to Penn she was just naturally very pretty with her near black hair, that soft accent and the innocence of her blushing. They all had taken a toll on him.

"Ever had lunch at "*PV*" in Portuguese Cove?" he asked before he realized what he had said.

"Penn, my Honda has over 100,000 miles and barely gets me to work. What's *PV* and where is Portuguese Cove?"

"Good. It'll be a surprise. My thanks for being the sunshine in my life today."

"But, don't you have a ...?"

"Oh, you mean a wife? That's OK, and a fair question. Probably overdue, too. The answer is both yes and no. I've been solo since we parted about a year ago. It started as a simple disagreement. Nothing, really. More on the scale of whether she liked chocolate and I like vanilla. But it had been brewing for a long time. I guess we never saw it coming.

Clearly my cancer was the catalyst. So one day she decided that spending the rest of her life with someone who has an incurable cancer was not doable and she left. Said I was toxic, too. That part was very cutting. For sure I never saw that coming.

I didn't hear from her for a long time. Then, she let me know in an email she had taken a job at a local office of her current employer and would be staying near her sister's in Charleston. Our intimacy has been reduced to short 'How are you?' emails about every four to six weeks, or so.

It's a long story, but the short version is that the relationship is over and has been for about a year.

I don't see any possibility of returning to our previous marriage. Don't want to, either. While we've lived apart for about a year now, in reality the time apart has made it possible for me to see how much we had been living together, but apart, long before she moved out. While my cancer was the catalyst of the separation, clearly any real intimacy had not been in the relationship for a long time.

In that sense I guess her decision to leave was actually best for both of us. Obviously, the cancer needed my commitment and she needed a way to say goodbye.

So I believe we are both better off to see the year apart as a good reality check to re-build our lives than to try to re-kindle something that belongs in the past. I've reached a place where soon I intend to suggest we make the separation permanent and amicable. Sorry for getting into my stuff, but I thought since you asked you should know the story."

"I'm glad you told me. But whatever anyone tells you, you are not toxic. No one can get your cancer and none of your drugs are a risk to anyone. Do you hear me? [as she gave his hand a gentle caress].

Someone else would be more at risk if you had a common cold than from either your cancer or the treatments we give you at the hospital," Sari said emphatically, but still under the influence of being tired and not yet the mocha's caffeine.

"Seriously? You mean that? I thought … I mean, like you know … like in an intimate relationship there would be risks," he said suddenly blushing as if caught in a news flash.

"Right, and no excuses. You're not a risk to anyone. The ZQT is a non-chemo targeted therapy and it's fully purged after about six hours and your cancer is now under control in your immune system."

"OK, but I have one more question. Am I still a tourist?" Penn asked because now he just had to know, but with a slight smile.

"I'm really sorry I said that to you. Can you forgive me?" she said defensively with another of her classic blushes.

Sensing how their relationship had deepened Penn side-stepped her question, "Sari, I really want you to stay. Please say yes."

Seeing him as someone she really wanted to trust Sari replied, "OK ... But I don't know where Portuguese Cove is and my car is kind of so-so. Did you walk here or do you have a car?"

"Mine is the black Porsche 911 behind me. Is it OK? I mean ..."

"Oh, yes ... uh, sure ... You never told me you had a Porsche convertible," Sari said [with a surprise smile] while looking over his shoulder at the car. But I am really tired ... are you still OK with ..."

"Sure. We'll put the top up and you can nap to some soft jazz. I've been looking for a non-solo reason to drive down to Portuguese Cove for lunch at *PV*. Are you OK with upscale Mexican, like ceviche with a chardonnay? Actually, we'll be there in time for the chardonnay to counteract your mocha. *PV's* sea bass ceviche is incredible with a chardonnay. Great view, too. Just nod once for yes."

Still dazed, Sari managed the single nod, but asked with a cautious smile, "Could you leave the top down?"

"Great. Let's put your Honda in the free-lot behind the community center and we'll be on our way."

Under way to Portuguese Cove he turned on the Porsche's audio system to Chris Botti's trumpet soft jazz "No Ordinary Love" and gave Sari a light grey blanket with the comment, "911's are not known for their B&B qualities. Here's a soft fuzzy so you can nap."

"Thanks. But you still didn't tell me what PV is and where is Portuguese Cove?" Sari asked, while looking amazed at the Porsche's beautiful red leather interior.

"Oops, you're right. I was distracted [looking at her with another smile]. The restaurant's name is "Puerto Vallarta", otherwise known as PV, a really neat Mexican restaurant on the water in Portuguese Cove. It's about 60 miles due south. I think you'll love it.

Besides, the Porsche already knows the way along the coast. We'll be there just after noon and we'll probably have the view to ourselves. Do you like the soft jazz ...?"

But he needn't have asked about the soft jazz, as Sari was soon asleep.

WIFM - Reality Assessment #14

"Imagine" ... We really can dent cancer's universe.

BP Score Card:
Ping = 0, Pong = 0, Penn = 3 – Never let cancer be a stop sign to
                                your life's happiness.
                              – Always be on the offense.
                              – Always be denting cancer's universe!

Epilogue

What a piece of work is man.

It's as true in cancer as in life,
as one chapter ends another always begins.

Ping: Rare as it is, some people just seem able to motor-on in defiance of all the rules. While it appears that Ping is doing so as the last chapter ends, it's an illusion.

Back in real life Ping still enjoyed a good cigar, the best bourbon and deep sea fishing while the successive treatments extracted higher and higher tolls. That is, he continued to ingest the same tobacco smoke and alcohol carcinogens into his urinary system to continue brewing his cancer. He endured the increasingly adverse symptoms and treatments as his price to enjoy the life he wanted, the way he wanted to live it. What more did his cancer need?

But, in truth, Ping was burning the candle at both ends as the treatments severely worsened and he reached the eventual conversation with his oncologist, "Sorry, but there is nothing more we can do for you. You should make sure your affairs are in order, and soon." As the saying goes, "He had seen the movie and he knew the ending". Ping was just determined to rewrite the in-between-scenes.

Pong: In this story Pong still has time. But in real life it's true and I could not, not tell the truth. Pong lost his battle against the melanoma, much like the story evolved, but soon after this story ended. In real life he did not develop a "Penn" to reach out to when he could and needed to most.

The melanoma likely began in him as a youth – due to too much sun exposure - and went undetected until it emerged as itchy sores on his back. By the time it was diagnosed as melanoma it had already metastasized. Mistakes made in diagnosing and treating the melanoma further cost valuable time and compounded the risks. Leaving him with precious little time, and none to waste.

How often have we heard this?

By the time he had finally enrolled in the clinical trial the end of his life was already being scripted by his melanoma. He just had not yet read the email. He was a good husband, a wonderful father and a true friend. Sadly, this should have never happened.

Mimi: Truly beautiful in every conceivable way. She was a person who loved life and was a wonderful wife, mom and my dearest friend. Losing a friend like Mimi to something so cruel, so senseless as cancer just stops us cold, gripped by pain in our hearts.

I guess I just don't get it because I still have no relief from the pain or an answer to the relentless question, Why?

Penn: Penn's cancer is not curable. It is nearly always fatal within the first two to three years from the onset of symptoms.

By applying his *My Chronic Cancer Advocacy,* strategy and tactics, Penn was able to reach a Mexican-standoff with the cancer.

Unbeknownst to him at the time he became a patient of Dr. Collins he already had eleven tumors, including two large tumors in his neck that were capable of rupturing at any time and three smaller tumors within a centimeter of his esophagus.

Absent his *My Chronic Cancer Advocacy* that produced Dr. Collins, Sari and the ZQT non-chemo-chemo at the cancer centric-hospital and Penn was to otherwise fulfill Dr. Childs' dire prediction. He would be dead in about six months – by his next and last birthday.

Penn became a survivor because he learned to accept his cancer as a serious life threat, to make *My Chronic Cancer* his strategic goal, to develop his own *My Cancer Advocacy* as his tactical means <u>and to honestly manage the accumulating information.</u>

Penn's cancer is a ruthlessly deadly adversary. But with these tools he has learned how to contain its spread and to minimize the adverse effects of the treatments. With his team he has regained his health and he has transitioned to a maintenance treatment plan that he follows religiously.

He has a new diet of seafood, poultry, vegetables, fruits and fluids. His alcohol intake is limited to wine and an occasional beer. He never smoked anything. He has reduced stress levels and he no longer chases materialism for the sake of materialism.

He is not home free, but he has done a good job of integrating the three legs of the three-legged stool: Resources, Technology and Penn.

There is no reason he cannot go-forward to live a long and otherwise normal life, albeit by faithfully observing his new maintenance plan. Penn is managing his cancer and his new reality well. It is no longer managing him. **Penn is fully on the offense against his cancer.**

Good job. Keep improving.

Yes, it can be done. You really can change certainty.

****

"Just One More Thing."

In truth, there were six of us cancer patients. Two with solid tumors and four with blood cancers. Only Penn knew all the other five. True-true friends.

Though only Penn survived, just as in the story in both books, his friends' lives live on. They live on through both books to make possible your own implementation of *My Chronic Cancer Advocacy*.

And, yes, there really is an *Un Bel Di*.

Table 1: Overview of Cancer Patient Experiences

Patient / Doctor		Practice	Diagnosis	Result
Ping	Dr. Abbott	PCP/OCP	Infection	Antibiotic
"	" "	"	Abdominal pain	Steroid pill
"	" "	"	Bladder cancer	Treatment plan
"	Dr. Allen	Oncology	Bladder cancer	Chemo & Radiation
Pong	Dr. Baker	PCP	Skin rash	Steroid ointment
"	Dr. Benson	Dermatology	Melanoma	Surgical removal
"	Dr. Bates	Oncology	Melanoma	Treatment plan
"	Local surgeon	Surgery	Melanoma	Surgery & biopsy
"	Dr. Black	Oncology	Melanoma	Treatment plan
"	Dr. Butts	Sp. Oncology	Melanoma	MM-013 clinic
"	Dr. Bernstein	SP. Oncology	Melanoma	Radiation
Penn	Dr. Cain	PCP	Lymphoma	None
"	Dr. Cannon	Surgeon	Sinus Infect.	Surgical biopsy
"	Dr. Carter	PCP	None	No opinion
"	Dr. Carlson	Infect. Disease	None	No opinion
"	Dr. Casey	Infect. Disease	None	No opinion
"	Dr. Cash	Dermatology	Unknown	Referral
"	Dr. Chan	ENT-Oncology	Cancer	Ref to Dr. Chase
"	Dr. Calli	Lyme Disease	None	No diagnosis
"	Dr. Chase	Oncology	NHL Lymph.	NHL lymphoma
"	Dr. Childs	Sp. Oncology	NHL Lymph.	Confirmed NHL
				Watch & See
				CsA clinical
"	Dr. Cho	Sp. Oncology	NHL Lymph.	CsA opinion
"	Dr. Clancy	Sp. Oncology	None	Not an option
"	Dr. Clark	Sp. Oncology	NHL Lymph.	P3 clinical
"	Dr. C.	Oncology	None	Resident to
				Dr. Clark
"	Dr. Collins	Sp. Oncology	NHL Lymph	NHL specialist

An interesting snapshot view of their journeys.
But who is really on the offense against their cancer?

Table 2: DNA-like Framework™ BP Score Card Summary

Chapter	Ping	Pong	Penn
---	0	1	16 – From *Cancer: Who Gave Me Cancer?*
1	0	0	1 – Resources, resources, resources
2	0	1	1 – Rebuild your diet for health
3	0	1	3 – Stay engaged and on the offense
			– Pay attention to inflection points
			– Evaluate your team
4	0	2	0 – Beware the educated heart
			– Heed the advice of others
5	0	0	2 – Build confidence in you team
			– My Chronic Advocacy, always
6	0	0	0 – Be aware of depression
			– Continue to build options
7	0	1	1 – The big picture is in the dots
8	0	0	1 – Build real heroes
9	0	0	1 – Be part of your feed-back loop
10	0	1	0 – Be open to new ideas
11	0	0	3 – Bad things happen in cancer
			– Cancer doesn't care
			– Keep moving
12	0	1	2 – Have an open awareness
			– Honestly accept changes
13	0	1	3 – Remission is not cancer free
			– Beware of fantasy
			– Nothing is impossible
14	0	0	3 – Cancer is not a stop sign
			– Always be on the offense
			– OK to dent cancer's universe
Total(s)	0	9	37

Look again at the message in their journeys. It's not just the bottom line score, but also the process. *"Imagine our audacity."*

It can happen when you are always on offense, but not on defense.

Credits

Cover Photo	National Cancer Institute (NCI), USA
	Rob Shickel
Dedications	*No Man is an Island*, John Donne
Introduction	Sir Winston Churchill
Prologue	*King Lear*, Wm. Shakespeare
Chapter 1	*Henry VI*, Wm. Shakespeare
Chapter 2	Michael Cope
Chapter 3	*The Bear*, William Faulkner
Chapter 4	*Sergeant Pepper*, The Beatles
Chapter 5	Joe Namath
Chapter 6	*Little Lies*, Fleetwood Mac
Chapter 7	*As You Like It*, Wm. Shakespeare
	Sari
Chapter 8	James Baldwin
Chapter 9	*Star Wars*, Master Yoda
Chapter 10	*Star Wars*, Luke
	Star Wars, Master Yoda
Chapter 11	Rob Shickel
	Time To Say Goodbye, Sarah Brightman
	Blade Runner, Ridley Scott & Phillip Dick
Chapter 12	*The Winter's Tale*, Wm. Shakespeare
Chapter 13	Old Chinese Proverb
Chapter 14	Steve Jobs
	If I Had a Hammer, Peter, Paul & Mary
	Feelings, Acker Bilk
	No Ordinary Love, Chris Botti
	Imagine, John Lennon
Epilogue	*Hamlet*, Wm. Shakespeare
	Rob Shickel
Just One	Steve Jobs
More Thing	*Madama Butterfly*, Giacomo Puccini
Table #2	Barak Obama

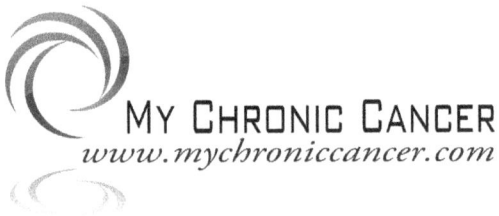

www.ingramcontent.com/pod-product-compliance
Lightning Source LLC
Chambersburg PA
CBHW031151270326
41931CB00006B/224